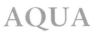

AQUA

Water Remedies
in Homeopathy

Saltire Books *Saltire Books Limited, Glasgow, Scotland*

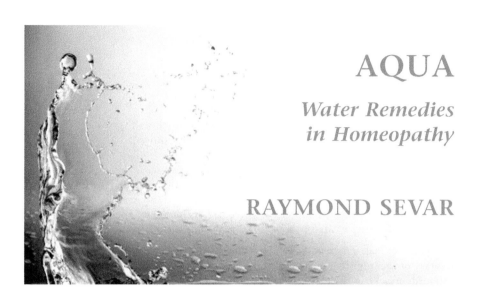

AQUA

Water Remedies
in Homeopathy

RAYMOND SEVAR

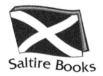

Saltire Books   *Saltire Books Limited, Glasgow, Scotland*

Published by Saltire Books Ltd

18–20 Main Street, Busby, Glasgow G76 8DU, Scotland
books@saltirebooks.com   www.saltirebooks.com

Cover, Design, Layout and Text © Saltire Books Ltd 2022

 is a registered trademark

First published in 2022

Typeset by Type Study, Scarborough, UK in 9¼ on 13½ Stone Serif
Printed and bound in the UK by TJ Books Ltd, Padstow, Cornwall

ISBN 978-1-908127-44-0

For Saltire Books
Project Development: Lee Kayne
Editorial: Steven Kayne
Design: Phil Barker
Index: Laurence Errington

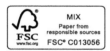

CONTENTS

DEDICATION

I dedicate this book to:

- My beloved wife Patricia, to whom I have been married for 42 years.
- My daughters Katherine, Helen and Clare – the light and joy of our lives.
- Our grandchildren April, Mila, Frederick and Elizabeth who are beyond all words.

ACKNOWLEDGEMENTS

I would like to thank:

- Steven and Lee Kayne of Saltire Books for their unfailing support and guidance from first draft to final.
- My medical doctors practising homeopathy for their care, understanding and compassion as well as some remarkable remedies especially Anton van Rhijn and Julie Geraghty.

ABOUT THE AUTHOR

Raymond Sevar is a Medical Doctor practising Homeopathy since 1993 in Carlisle, Cumbria. He has presented lectures and seminars in Scotland, Japan, India, Russia, USA, Portugal, Poland and Germany.

He was Dean of the Faculty of Homeopathy from 2005 to 2012 and continues on the Examiners Board. He is involved in peer supervision and has directed two homeopathic provings – the 1st proving of the water of the Cross Spring in Bath is part of this book.

PREFACE

The purpose of this book is to present the waters used in homeopathy as a coherent family of mineral remedies with their own themes, sensations and keywords in a form which will be useful in homeopathic clinical practice. The basic themes of the Aqua were first described by Alicia Hay[1] and form a firm foundation for this work. Alicia, a professional homeopath from New Zealand, did start to write a book on the waters but stopped after writing mind maps for 19 waters.

My interest in the waters as homeopathic remedies began with my struggles to understand the children for whom I first prescribed *Aqua Sanicula* in the 1990s.[2]

In 2000 the British Homeopathic Congress was held in Bath where I presented my homeopathic proving of the water of the Cross Spring in Bath, *Aqua Bath*.[3]

My proving was followed by some incredibly rich springs (notably *Aqua Hochstein*) and river waters (especially *Aqua Taosca*) and manmade waters (and a surprise – distilled water *Aqua Destillata*), helped me form a clearer understanding of the Aqua.

In 2005 I met with David Warkentin who was developing his vision of MacRepertory and Reference Works to enable study of families of homeopathic remedies to aid more accurate prescribing. We looked at the spring waters and found an old and well-established group of remedies which were forgotten and neglected.[4]

Almost 20 years in the writing ... gathering information on each Aqua, gathering rubrics together in Clinical Rubric Clusters, Useful and/or Unusual Rubrics ... enables synthesis – seeing related single remedies, then related remedy families.

Other information sources include Complete Repertory.[5]

Nomenclature in Aqua remedies

The 'Aqua' are homeopathic medicines with their own themes, sensations, key words, clinical symptom clusters, rubrics and clinical indications. The nomenclature of the 'Aqua' should be consistent with the current nomenclature of mineral remedies. In this work the name of each of the waters begins with 'Aqua' (also after name in Index). I would suggest that the repertory abbreviations are changed to begin each with aq-.

The current names of the waters more often begin with the name of the site of the spring e.g., Narzan 'aqua' or the ancient name of the water in the native language e.g. Skookum Chuck 'aqua' and the repertory abbreviations reflect this.

Many 'Aqua' are well established old remedies but tend to be forgotten or overlooked during case analysis and reperatorisation. The repertories list remedy abbreviations alphabetically. During case taking and analysis when we look at relevant rubrics the 'Aqua' are scattered throughout the rubric. A change in nomenclature to begin the name of each water with 'Aqua' and the repertory abbreviations with 'aq-' would gather the remedies together in rubrics, emphasise their preponderance within certain rubrics and repertory graphs and aid us in the choice of an 'Aqua' as the best remedy for more patients. Such a change in nomenclature would have implications for those who write repertories and homeopathic software programs and homeopathic pharmacies in their listing of remedies.

Raymond Sevar
Carlisle, Cumbria
31st October 2021

References

1   Lee A. *Homeopathic Mind Maps – Vol. 2, Mineral Kingdom.* Auckland: Moozoonsii Publishing, 2010, pp 87–111.
2   Sevar, R., *Sanicula aqua*: three clinical cases and a heuristic. *Homeopathy*, 2005; **94**: 125–131.
3   Sevar, R. The water of the Cross Spring in Bath – a Homeopathic Proving Homeopathic Links. 2002; **15**(3): 183–188.
4   MacRepertory of Kent Homeopathic Software written and developed by David Warkentin and now known as Synergy Homeopathic.
5   van Zandvoort, R. *Comparative Repertory.* Leidsschhendam NL: Institute for Research in Homeopathic Information and Symptomatology, 1994.

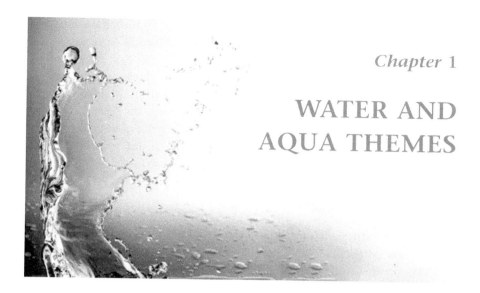

Chapter 1

WATER AND
AQUA THEMES

Imagine our world 100 years after every one of us insisted that the first priority of governments is the provision of free clean drinking water. I dare you, take a moment and imagine. Water permeates our bodies, our language, our cultures, our religions, our poetry and fiction and our conversations.

Water is essential to life

Every living thing on our planet contains water and requires water to complete its life cycle. Our human bodies are 65–75% by weight water. We need to drink water to live and if we stop drinking water we die. The availability of clean drinking water is the single most important contributing factor to the rise in health and increased life expectancy of the human race – more important than any influence of medicine, even mass immunisation.

Water is the most precious natural resource of our planet

Our best estimate is that the Earth contains 326 million cubic miles of water. The earth is a fairly closed system – it loses or gains very little water – the same water that existed on the earth millions of years ago is still present today. The overall weight of our planet's biomass has also remained almost constant over time – evolution and meteor impacts have changed the relative preponderance of species – 2/3rds of the total biomass lives in water and 1/3rd lives on dry land. Water covers 70–75% of the surface of the planet – more than half the volume of fresh water is stored underground in aquifers and in the polar icecaps. The water cycle drives our weather. We are all taught the water cycle at school. The heat of the sun causes water to evaporate from the oceans, lakes and rivers and rise through the air as water vapour which collects as clouds. In due time the clouds cool and deposit the water as rain, sleet, hail or snow.

Water and thirst

Water is a colourless, odourless and tasteless liquid, yet we can see it and smell it and taste it. We are drawn to water, to walk beside water, to picnic and play beside or in water. For many of us it boosts our energy and mood and being at the sea or sea bathing can ameliorate our suffering when we are ill. For others, symptoms can be aggravated by wet weather, or by becoming wet and chilled. Living with a chronic illness entails carrying a certain burden of suffering despite the best treatment. Many people are able to endure a surprising degree of pain or itching yet the sensation of thirst will not be denied – it intrudes into our consciousness and grows until we must drink to quench our thirst.

Reverence for Water

Water has been held in reverence by all the peoples of our planet from ancient times. The sacramental use of water continues in our ancient and modern religions. Since the industrial revolution our use of water and attitudes to water have changed significantly. We have polluted our atmosphere and water cycle so much that we appear to have caused a change in our climate. All over the planet we endure more extreme weather with greater swings in temperatures. The polar ice caps continue to melt as never before. Many parts of the world now experience deluges of rain falling in a short time resulting in serious flooding – most of Cumbria and the south of Scotland were flooded in 2015.

Purity of Water

There is no such thing as pure water – all water contains something other than water. Water contains oxygen from the air – the colder the water is the more oxygen can dissolve in it. Water also contains the other gases in air: nitrogen, carbon dioxide, traces of the noble gases. Even purified pharmacy grade water (Purified Water B.P.) and distilled water contain traces of other substances. Given enough time water will begin to dissolve almost everything. Whatever water is stored in, water will begin to dissolve its surface – if stored in glass it will contain traces of silica. The elements of column 10 of the Periodic Table – Carbon, Silicon, Nickel, Palladium, Gadolinium, Platinum and Curium – resists the longest yet even a diamond will eventually begin to lose mass as some dissolves into water.

Constituents of water

Water molecules are composed of two atoms of hydrogen and one atom of oxygen – H_2O. It is naturally radioactive.

Hydrogen

Hydrogen was first distinguished as an element in 1766 by Henry Cavendish and named by Lavoisier in 1781. The name is from the Greek – "hydro" meaning water and "genes" meaning forming. Hydrogen is the most abundant element in the universe – estimated at 90% of all atoms and ¾ of the mass of the universe and makes up about 0.75% by weight of the Earth's crust. It is the energy and fuel of suns which through nuclear fusion of two Hydrogen atoms make Helium and eventually every other element. Hydrogen is an extremely light gas – the only element that can escape Earth's gravity.

Hydrogen exists as 3 isotopes (3 in 1, Trinity).

- Ordinary Hydrogen has one proton and one electron.
- Deuterium has one neutron, one proton and one electron – it is radioactive.
- Tritium has two neutrons, one proton and one electron – it is radioactive and releases a beta particle.

Before the explosion of the first hydrogen bomb the natural Tritium concentrations in water was 0–10 Tritium Units (TU). Afterwards the levels rose to 6000TU in rainfall over Europe. The water cycle since has mixed all this Tritium with the world's water. Only the water deep in glaciers now has the original concentration of Tritium.

Hydrogen is the first element formed in the unfolding of creation. In the Periodic Table of Elements, it is naturally in Row 1, Column 1.

From Dr Jan Scholten's Themes and Key words of Hydrogen:[1]

Row 1: Column 1:

- Start, begin, initiate, impulsive, instinctive, spontaneous and unpredictable.
- One, one-sided, single, single-minded, sole, alone, lonely.
- Being, whole, just, true or untrue.
- Naive, childish, unborn.
- Space, time.
- Simple, simpleton, thoughtless, fool, psychosis.

Oxygen

Oxygen, atomic number 8, in water is covalently bonded to 2 atoms of hydrogen.

From Dr Scholten's Themes and Key words of Oxygen.[2]

Row 2:

- I, individual, person, body, child, hero.
- Life, value, meaning, self-worth.
- Ethical: good and bad, lust, possessions.
- Magic and myths.

Column 16:

- Rest, reconcile, deepening, memory.
- Past, lost, over, outcast.
- Neglect, decay, ruin, rags, lazy, philosophy, fantasy.
- Rotten, ugly, foul, offensive, putrid, disgust.
- Asking, begging, luring, tempting.

Water Words are Aqua Words

We all use words to do with weather and water – these are water cycle words – we do not notice we do. Our patients also use water/aqua words and we edit them out without noticing that we do so. Patients who need an Aqua remedy use Aqua words much more often than others and we do not register the words as significant. Those of us who video cases will hear them on replay but may still not realise the significance of their frequency.

111 Water and Aqua Words

Listed below are 111 words about water, what water is, what water does, what water means to us.

Liquid, fluid, wet, condensation, damp, dew.
Freezing, frost, ice, glacier.
Melting, evaporating, vapour, drop, cloud.
Drizzle, shower, rain, deluge, hail, fog, mist, snow, snowflake.

Flow, turbulent, trickle, torrent, river, stream, spate, flood.
Current, whirlpool, sea, ocean, tide, ripple, wave, tsunami.
Reflection, puddle, lake, oasis.

Resilience, bubble, simmer, boil, steam.
Seep, permeate, dissolve, dilute, erode, corrosion.
Buoyant, floating, sinking, drowning.
Washing, bathing, splashing, swimming.
Gurgling, gushing, geyser.

Clear, clarity, crystal, pure, spring.
Sparkling, pellucid, rainbow.
Starlit, moonlit, sunlit.

Clean, fresh, stale, stagnant, effluent, sewage.
Still, calm, neutral, surface, tension.
Deep, shallow.
Thirst, refreshing, hydration, dehydration.
Dousing, diviner, intuition.
Passing, birth, life.
Reverence, holy, sacred, sacrament, baptism, repentance, absolution.
Form, pattern, memory, radioactive.

Aqua Words and Levels in Case Taking and Analysis

Level 1: Name

• Liquid, rain, snow, ice.

Level 2: Symptom

• Wet, melting, evaporating, freezing, simmering, boiling.

Level 3: Emotion

• Calm, buoyant, turbulent, whirlpool, torrent.

Level 4: Delusion

• Corrosion, cloud, iceberg, glacier, ocean.

Level 5: Vital Sensation

• Flow, bubble, glass, bubble in glass.

Water/Aqua words and Miasms

Acute – extreme, panic, life or death:

- Flooding, drowning, tsunami.

Typhoid – urgency, risk of death but recover with effort:

- Riptide, deluge, flash-flood.

Psora – struggle and effort, lifelong, discomfort, hope, stuck:

- Freezing, melting, snowing, drizzle, shower, rain, trickle, paddling, swimming.

Ringworm – trying and giving up:

- Ebb and flow; evaporating.

Malaria – stuck and harassed:

- Turbulent, torrent, sinking.

Sycosis – fixed, avoid, hidden, accept:

- Glacier, iceberg, aquifer, puddle, fog, mist, moat.

Cancer – control, perfection, lifelong effort beyond endurance:

- Clear, clarity, crystal, pure, spring, sparkling, pellucid, rainbow, snowflake.
- Current, reflection, still, calm, neutral, buoyant.
- Reverence, repentance, absolution.

Tubercular – oppression, suffocation, hectic activity to break free, burn-out, bleeding:

- Simmer, boil, pressure, gushing, geyser.

Leprosy – despised, cast out, unclean:

- Stale, stagnant, bog, effluent, sewage.

Syphilis – hopeless despair, degeneration, destruction:

- Erosion, corrosion, dissolved, evaporated.

A.I.D.S. – contamination through barriers:

- Seep, permeate, contaminate.

Aqua Themes, Sensations and Keywords

Water, like everything else, is more than the sum of its parts. Each Aqua remedy brings something unique from its form, content, pattern and memory yet the Aqua embrace all that water is to form a coherent family of mineral remedies.

Vital Sensations – Flow and Bubble

Flow

- Effortless.
- Easy.
- Flowing downhill.
- Flowing like a river, flowing around bends.

Bubble

- In a glass bubble.
- Bubble frozen in glass – can't move, can't flow.
- Bubble stuck in stomach – can't burp.
- Lots of bubbles fizzing together.

Aqua Themes and Keywords and Sensations *as if*

Clear and clean and pure and bright

- DREAMS; light (11): *amet.*, aq-des., coff., *galeoc-c.*, kola., lach., mus-m., nept-m., perla, ratt-n., uv-lux.

Intuition and imagination

- INTUITIVE (14): acon., *amet.*, aq-hoch., aquilr-a., bar-c., cann-i., ilx-p., lac-leo., plut-n., pras-c., pras-o., sep., spect., terb.

Sensitivity and vulnerability: emotional and cognitive – loss of resilience – overwhelm

Remembering the past and being unable to move on – ongoing emotional pain

Unable to: reflect dispassionately; gain closure from relationships; let go of the past.

- RESERVED; partner, towards (2): aq-hoch., haliae-lc.
- RESERVED; displeasure (6): aq-mar., **Aur.**, **Ign.**, **Ip.**, **Nat-m.**, **Staph.**
- FAMILY, aversion to; parents; mother (6): alum-s., aq-taosc., niob., **Posit.**, *scorp.*, **Thuj.**

Suppression of Emotions – Sublimation of Libido

Fear to look too deeply at emotions:

- DETACHED; relationships, from emotional (5): aq-hoch., erb., iod., lute., stan-e.
- DETACHED; family, home, from (8): aq-hoch., coriand., erb., heli., iod., lute., *pot-a.*, stan-e.

Desire to Beget Children and Be a Parent

Children – great love for children – dreams of children.

- PREGNANT, desire to be (3): aq-des., brachy-s-p., onc-t.
- CHILDREN; desires to; have, to beget, to nurture (8): aq-des., aq-taosc., lim-b-c., lsd, nat-m., *onc-t.*, ox-ac., *plac.*
- CHILDLESS, ailments from being (10): aq-des., aq-taosc., aur., lac-h., lim-b-c., lsd, nat-m., *onc-t.*, ox-ac., plac.

Abdomen

- MOVEMENTS; foetus, as of; first movement (1): aq-carl.
- MOVEMENTS; foetus, as of (16): aq-carl., bacch-a., cinis-p., con., conv., **Croc.**, latex, *leon.*, **Nat-c.**, sabin., sals-t., stann., **Sulph.**, tarent., **Ther.**, THUJ.

Sensation as if of time long past

- Sensation as if of past people and past places.
- Sensation as if of past life – of being someone else – of living long ago.

- DREAMS; World; he is moving in a new (7): aq-taosc., borrel., camph., corv-c., lar-ar., lsd, oplo-h.
- DREAMS; time (11): acan-pl., aq-mar., bamb-a., c-di-o., cyg-b., helod-c., lsd, *onc-t.*, rhus-g., sang., telo-s.

Sensation of isolation and detachment

- Looking at the world through a glass window.
- Separated from the world.
- Locked inside another world.
- Of loneliness yet desire to be alone.

Water

- Thirst for water.
- Watering from eyes, nose, vaginal discharge, moisture from anus.

- Dreams of water: floods, swimming, bathing, drowning, dead body in the sea.
- Dryness: mucous membranes and skin.

Exhaustion – extreme and persistent

- Physical – must lie down.
- Mental – poor concentration and hard to read or write.

Sensitivity and vulnerability: emotional and cognitive – loss of resilience – overwhelm

Sensitivity and vulnerability yet functioning well

- QUICK to act; waking, on (3): *aq-hoch.*, *lac-h.*, lac-mat.
- MIRTH, hilarity, liveliness; morning; waking, on (2): aq-carl., chin.
- MUSIC; desires; compose, to (2): aq-hoch., pras-o.
- DREAMS; control; being in (3): aq-mar., lac-cpr., *sol.*
- DREAMS; Peaceful (9): aq-taosc., coriand., *cyg-c.*, haliae-lc., hippo-k., lac-eq., *mand.*, nux-m., spig.

- DELUSIONS, imaginations; runs; never before, she can run like (2): agar., aq-taosc.
- SELFLESSNESS (9): anh., aq-mar., arn., iod., lant-o., nat-c., puls., rhus-t., staph.
- PAIN; aggravates; emotional, of others (4): aq-carl., dysp-n., erb., lim-b-c.
- SADNESS; others, for (10): apei-s., aq-mar., ars., cocc., **Dros.**, hep., neod-c., phos., rhus-t., sulph.
- SELF-SUFFICIENT (12): aq-mar., calc., des-ac., erb-s., ferr-ma., gado., gins., mag-c., neod-o., neod-p., terb-s., ulm-c.

Loss of resilience

- TELEVISION watching; desires (3): *adon.*, aq-hoch., lac-as.
- COMPUTERS, electronic games; desires (6): *aq-hoch.*, calc-i., euro-n., excr-can., thul., ytte-p.

- EXCITEMENT, excitable; morning; rising, on (3): *aloe*, aq-carl., iber.
- ANXIETY; motion; ameliorates; fast (2): aq-mar., saroth.
- ANXIETY; afternoon; ameliorates (2): aq-mar., tab.
- ANXIETY; drinks, cold, ameliorate; ice cold (2): agar-em., aq-mar.

- FEAR; change, of (2): *aq-skook.*, med.
- FEAR; looked at, when (10): aq-mar., *ars.*, bar-c., calc., germ., med., meli., ratt-n., rhus-t., tub.

- OBSTINATE, headstrong; night (2): aq-sanic., dig.
- QUARRELSOMENESS, scolding; family, with her; husband, to (7): *amet.*, *aq-hoch.*, calop-s., haliae-lc., hyos., lac-lup., **Thuj.**

Overwhelm

- DREAMS; spied on, of being (2): aq-mar., neon
- DREAMS; Hopeless (4): acan-pl., aids, aq-mar., lac-lox-a.
- ANGUISH; night; waking, on (4): aq-kiss., kali-br., **Nat-s.**, **Nux-v.**
- ANGUISH; menses; before (5): aq-carl., cocc., **Graph.**, **Murx.**, stann.
- ANXIETY; constriction, with; chest, of; convulsive, spasmodic (2): aq-carl., **Cupr.**
- BESIDE oneself, being; trifles, about (4): **Aq-Carl.**, dros., kres., thuj.

- CHAOTIC; life (4): *aq-hoch.*, neod-c., *plut-n.*, pras-m.
- DRESS, dresses; indecently (8): aq-mar., ephe., **Hell.**, herin., **Hyos.**, salx-f., sec., **Stram.**
- INDIFFERENCE, apathy; opinion of others, of (9): agath-a., androc., aq-taosc., bufo, falco-p., neod-f., *stoi-k.*, tax., ulm-c.

- BROODING; cares, worries, unpleasant things (6): aq-kiss., **Aur.**, **Ign.**, nitro., ros-g., staph.
- SUICIDAL disposition; love disappointment, from (8): ant-c., aq-hoch., **Aur.**, **Bell.**, **Caust.**, **Hyos.**, plut-n., **Staph.**
- RAGE, fury; malicious (11): aq-taosc., **Bell.**, cann-s., choc., cocc., cupr., lyc., mosch., neon, petr., sec.

Suppression of Emotions and Sublimation of libido

- Chest; ANXIETY; mammae (2): aq-des., **PHOS.**
- Abdomen; MURMURING, muttering (2): *aq-carl.*, sabad.
- Abdomen; EMPTINESS, faintness; gnawing (3): aq-wild., hema-h., **Ox-ac.**
- Abdomen; TENSION; diaphragm (5): act-sp., **Aq-Carl.**, coch., coloc., sel.
- Back; TENSION; short, as if muscles too (5): aq-sanic., aur., hyos., lyc., sulph.
- Abdomen; RETRACTION; convulsive, spasmodic (9): aq-kiss., *act-sp.*, *chel.*, *plat.*, plb., plb-chr., stram., **Sul-ac.**, *tab.*

- FANCIES; lascivious; day and night (3): aq-taosc., chin., dig.
- Male; ERECTIONS; causeless (7): **Am-c.**, anac., aq-carl., ferr., ox-ac., sil., tarax.
- FANCIES; lascivious; tormenting (14): aq-mar., aster., bani-c., canth., coca, con., galeoc-c., graph., med., ozone, **Staph.**, stram., syph., tarent.

References

1 Scholten J. *Homeopathy and the Elements*. Utrecht: Stichting Alonissos, 2004. pp. 74–76.
2 *Ibid.*, pp. 175, 189, 203, 304, 513.

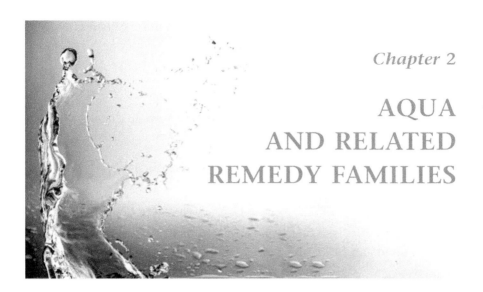

Chapter 2

AQUA
AND RELATED
REMEDY FAMILIES

Remedies and remedy families may be related in several ways:

- Share similar constituent minerals or plant alkaloids.
- Share a single or several emotional or physical symptoms or rubrics – Share and Compare.
- Share symptom or rubric clusters in 1 or more clinical disorders.
- Share similar general or local modalities.
- Share keywords or themes or sensations.

Degrees of relationship will be reflected in:

- The number of rubrics which contain both remedies.
- The concordance of general symptoms and modalities.
- The concordance of emotional and cognitive symptoms and rubrics.

The most closely related remedy families to the Aqua are:

- Fishes.
- Energy remedies – also called the Imponderables.
- Minerals: Gemstones, Gases, Acids and Lanthanides.
- Other animals: Milks and other Sarcodes, Birds and Ocean Invertebrates.
- Plants: Asteraceae.
- Multiple Shared Clinical Rubric Clusters: Coniferae, Liliaceae and.
- Solanaceae.

Comparison of two examples of Shared Clinical Rubric Clusters of
Aqua Sanicula with Sepia and Carbo animalis

Aqua Sanicula and Chloasma Gravidarum

Face

- YELLOW; saddle across; cheeks (4): aq-sanic., **Carb-an.**, ictod., **SEP.**
- YELLOW; saddle across; nose (8): aq-sanic., carb-an., chel., lyc., op., **SEP.**, sulph., tril.
- SADDLE across nose (10): aq-sanic., **Carb-an.**, chel., ictod., lyc., op., **SEP.**, sulph., syph., tril.
- BROWN; nose (8): aq-sanic., **Aur.**, **Carb-an.**, **Lyc.**, **Op.**, **SEP.**, **Sulph.**, **Syph.**

Aqua Sanicula and Prolapse Uterus

Share and Compare: Sepia officinalis, Murex purpurea and Lilium tigrinum.

Female

- PROLAPSE; uterus; standing; aggravates (4): aq-sanic., **Lappa**, nit-ac., **Sep.**
- PAIN; uterus; pressure; ameliorates; vulva, on (5): **Aq-Sanic.**, bell., lil-t., murx., sep.
- PAIN; uterus; supports abdomen with hands (9): aq-sanic., **Bell.**, fic-mac., helon., lat-h., **LIL-T.**, lyc., **Murx.**, **Sep.**

- PAIN; bearing down; uterus:
- Pressing on vulva ameliorates (5): **Aq-Sanic.**, **Bell.**, **LIL-T.**, **MURX.**, **SEP.**
- Pressure ameliorates (7): **Aq-Sanic.**, **Bell.**, ign., **LIL-T.**, mag-c., **MURX.**, **SEP.**
- Supports abdomen with hands (8): aq-sanic., **Bell.**, fic-mac., lat-h., **LIL-T.**, lyc., **Murx.**, **Sep.**
- Lying; ameliorates (9): **Agar.**, aq-sanic., aur-m-n., cimic., ign., onos., pall., podo., **Sep.**
- Rest; ameliorates (9): **Agar.**, aq-sanic., aur-m-n., cimic., ign., onos., pall., podo., **Sep.**

Aqua and Gemstones

Aqua and gemstones have common keywords and themes.

Keywords

- Clear, crystal, pure, precious, light and dark.

Themes

- Emotional sensitivity and vulnerability and suppression.

All rubrics containing a gemstone are gemstone triturates.

The gemstone immersion remedies of Peter Tumminello[1] are, to my mind, man-made Aqua remedies. Made by immersing a gemstone in a glass bowl of distilled water plus exposure to sunlight and moonlight, they will contain something of Aqua Destillata and Sol and Luna plus each gemstone, yet each will be more than the sum of their parts. Please refer to Peter's excellent works for detail.[1]

All gemstones except for diamond, amber and pearl arise from waters containing the requisite minerals in the correct proportions subjected to ferocious heat and enormous pressure. Pure carbon as graphite subjected to ferocious heat and enormous pressure results in a diamond. The remedy made from amber is called Succinum – is different. It is the sticky, resinous sap of an ancient conifer – this is why amber often contains an insect. Pearls are made by oysters or mussels as layers of calcium carbonate around a central tiny grain of silica which has penetrated the mollusc's muscle.

Aqua Hochstein and Gemstone and Milk and Energy and Lanthanides

- INTUITIVE (14): acon., *amet.*, aq-hoch., aquilr-a., bar-c., cann-i., ilx-p., lac-leo., plut-n., pras-c., pras-o., sep., spect., terb.

Aqua Hochstein and Gemstone and Rose

- DREAMS; Relationships (4): aq-hoch., lap-be-e., *ros-ca.*, soph-m.

Aqua Hochstein and Gemstone and Bird and Milk

- QUARRELSOMENESS, scolding; family, with his; husband, to (7): *amet.*, *aq-hoch.*, calop-s., haliae-lc., hyos., lac-lup., Thuj.

Aqua Marina and Gemstone and Rose

- DREAMS; Romantic (12): *am-c.*, aq-mar., blatta, bung-f., coco-n., junc., Kali-c., lam-cy., lap-be-e., lsd, *ros-ca-a.*, tax-br.

Aqua Carlsbad and Gemstone and Bird and Rose

- DREAMS; Grief (10): all-c., alum., *amet.*, aq-carl., arist-cl., *ars.*, caust., *cyg-c.*, ros-g., stront-c.

Aqua and Diamond

Face

- SENSITIVENESS; eyebrows (2): adam., aq-wild.
- FROWNING; sensation (3): adam., aq-franz., *enal-c.*

Mouth

- PAIN: Palate; Morning; waking, on (2): adam., aq-mar.

Chest

- PAIN; stitching; needles, as from; mammae; right (2): adam., aq-tep.

Aqua and Amber

- DREAMS; boars, pigs (4): aq-des., merl., succ., uv-lux.
- DREAMS; trees, of; chopping down (5): aq-des., cordy-a., lac-eq., stoi-k., succ.

Generalities

- BATHING, washing; aggravates; hair (3): aq-taosc., succ., tarent.

Aqua and Lanthanides

Keywords
Lanthanide[2]: autonomy, self, light, shadow, reflection, searching, deep, immune, auto-immune diseases.

Aqua and Lanthanide keywords in common:

- Light and shadow.
- Deep.
- Reflection and intuition.
- Sympathy and compassion and grief.

Aqua Marina and Lanthanides

- GRIEF; resigned (4): aq-mar., clem., erb., erb-o.
- SELFLESSNESS (9): anh., aq-mar., arn., iod., lant-o., nat-c., puls., rhus-t., staph.
- SADNESS; others, for (10): apei-s., aq-mar., ars., cocc., **Dros.**, hep., neod-c., phos., rhus-t., sulph.

Aqua Hochstein and Lanthanides

- MUSIC; desires; compose, to (2): aq-hoch., pras-o.
- COMPUTERS, electronic games; desires (6): *aq-hoch.*, calc-i., euro-n., excr-can., thul., ytte-p.

- DIVORCE, ailments from, aggravates; children, in (10): aeth., *aq-hoch.*, cer-
- c., cycl., dysp-n., excr-can., holm-o., lant-c., lant-o., nat-m.

Aqua Hochstein and 2 Lanthanides

- CHAOTIC; life (4): *aq-hoch.*, neod-c., *plut-n.*, pras-m.

Aqua Hochstein and 4 Lanthanides and Sarcode

- DISCORDS aggravate, ailments from; relatives, friends, between; parents (12): acon., Ant-t., *aq-hoch.*, bufo, chr., gado-n., gado-p., holm., lant-c., plac., *plut-n.*, prot.

Aqua Carlsbad and 2 Lanthanides

- PAIN; aggravates; emotional, of others (4): aq-carl., dysp-n., erb., lim-b-c.

Aqua and Sarcodes

Keywords of Sarcodes
- Function – perfect – normal.
- Balance and control.
- Order and limit and feedback.
- Flow and boundaries.
- Comfort zone.
- Connection and disconnection.

Keywords of Matridonal Sarcodes
- Identity, individual, potential, realization, awareness, awakening, recognition.
- Rebirth, incarnation, journey, acceptance, letting go, cutting ties.
- A journey to reconnect, to remember, to reform, to reclaim our identity, our.

Keywords and themes shared by Aqua and Sarcodes
- Flow and boundaries.

Aqua theme "Desire to Beget Children and be a Parent" is shared by Placenta humana.

Aqua and Milks

Rubric examples of an Aqua with 12 milks: Lac Humanum, Lac Maternum, Lac Asinum, Lac Equinum, Lac Caprinum, Lac Delphinum, Lac Leoninum,

Lac Loxodonta Africana, Lac Vaccinum Defloratum, Lac Cameli Dromedari and Lac Caninum.

Aqua Hochstein and Milks

- WEANING, ailments from (2): aq-hoch., lac-h.
- QUICK to act; waking, on (3): *aq-hoch., lac-h.,* lac-mat.
- TELEVISION watching; desires (3): *adon.,* aq-hoch., lac-as.
- DREAMS; Money; problems, with (3): aq-hoch., hema-h., lac-eq.
- DREAMS; Surgery, of (4): aq-hoch., lac-del., lac-leo., musca-d.

Aqua Marina and Milks

- DREAMS; Control; being in (3): aq-mar., lac-cpr., *sol.*
- DREAMS; Hopeless (4): acan-pl., aids, aq-mar., lac-lox-a.
- TIME; timelessness (14): aq-mar., ara-m., brachy-s-p., cann-i., clad-r., cyg-c., lac-lox-a., lap-c-b., *lsd,* mobil-ph., neon, onc-t., spect., tax.
- EAT, eating; more than she should (11): abies-c., aq-mar., **Ars.,** bacch-a., carc., eug., helod-c., lac-del., merc-v., onc-t., thul.

Aqua Sanicula and Milks

- DELUSIONS, imaginations; clothing, clothes; wet, is (9): **Aq-Sanic., Calc., Guai., Lac-d., Lyc., Phos., Ran-b., Sep., Verat-v.**

Perspiration

- STAINING; wash off, difficult to, indelible (4): aq-sanic., **Lac-d., Mag-c., Merc.**

Female

- PAIN; cramping; menses; before (5): aq-sanic., bute-j., lac-dr., stront-c., vanil.

Fever, heat

- INTENSE heat, 39+ C.; night (8): aq-sanic., **Ars.,** bac., chel., dor., lac-d., lachn., **Mag-c.**

Key to sarcodes other than milks – remedy abbreviations:

- Placenta humana = plac. Folliculinum = foll.
- DNA desoxyribose nucleic acid = des-ac and RNA Ribonucleic acid = rib-ac.
- Pituitary anterior = pit-a. Thyroidinum = thyr. Adrenaline = adren.
- Corticotropinum (ACTH) = cortico Cortisonum (Hydrocortisone) = cortiso.
- Adenosine tri-phosphate = atp.

- Atropine = Atropinum purum = atro.
- Oleum animale aethereum dippeli = ol-an – a distillation from deer antlers – an expression of testosterone plus the desire to beget children and be a parent.
- Ambra grisea – a natural secretion of the sperm whale – aromatic long chain alcohols.

Aqua and Sarcodes other than Milks

- DREAMS; cats, felines; wild (3): aq-hoch., ozone, *plac.*

Generalities

- TINGLING, prickling; heated, on becoming (2): aq-hoch., atp.

Sleep

- YAWNING; sitting, while (9): aq-carl., atro., bor., clem., cocc., nat-c., nicc., tarax., *viol-t.*

Ears

- PAIN; bathing, washing; aggravates (3): *aq-hoch.*, aq-taosc., cortico.

Mouth

- SALIVATION; cotton, like (6): aq-mar., bell., **Berb.**, **Nux-m.**, **Ol-an.**, **PULS.**

Heart and circulation

- PALPITATION heart; trembling, with; hands, of (6): acan-pl., am-c., aq-lipp., **Bov.**, elaps, thyr.

Female

- HYPERTROPHY, uterus (7): ant-i., aq-wies., **AUR.**, **Con.**, euph-pu., foll., ust.

Urine

- FISHY odour (11): abrom-aug., **Aq-Sanic.**, astac., bufo, conv., **Nat-c.**, **OL-AN.**, posit., uran., **Uran-n.**, vanil.

Extremities

- PAIN; sore, bruised; hands; left (3): aq-sanic., pitu-a., succ.
- INFLAMMATION; hands; palms (4): aq-skook., bry., m-arct., pitu-a.
- NUMBNESS, insensibility; upper limbs; carrying a load, from (3): **Ambr.**, aq-carl., sep.

Back

- PAIN; lumbar region, lumbago; lying; ameliorates; side, on (4): aq-sanic., des-ac., nat-s., zinc.

Aqua and Birds

Whooper Swan = cyg-c. Raven = corv-c. Bald Eagle = haliae-lc. Peregrine falcon = falco-p. Ara Macaw = ara-m. Californian Roadrunner = geoc-c. Herring Gull – lar-ar. Red Tailed Hawk – bute-j. Turkey Vulture – cath-a.

Related levels

- Sensitive to the suffering of others and compassionate.
- Desire to be a parent and nurture children.

In the birds there is the sense that when (as soon as) the children are grown up it is enough, and it is time for them to leave and fend for themselves.

Aqua Marina and Birds

- DREAMS; amorous; advances, unwanted (2): aq-mar., cyg-c.
- ANXIETY; talking; ameliorates (2): aq-mar., cyg-c.
- DELUSIONS, imaginations; Legs; cut off, are (8): aq-mar., bapt., **Bar-c.**, corv-c., halo., lsd, **Stram.**, tarent.
- TIME; timelessness (14): aq-mar., ara-m., brachy-s-p., cann-i., clad-r., cyg-c., lac-lox-a., lap-c-b., *lsd*, neon, onc-t., spect., tax. = 2 birds and 2 milks and salmon and gas.

Face

- DRYNESS; lips; night (7): ant-c., aq-mar., calad., calc-i., cham., *cyg-c.*, methylp-h.

Rectum

- DIARRHOEA; seashore, at (6): aq-mar., **Ars.**, bry., corv-c., **Syph.**, vip.

Aqua Sanicula and Birds

- FORGETFULNESS; Details, for (3): aq-sanic., cadm., falco-p.
- ANGER; touch aggravates (9): **Ant-c.**, **Aq-Sanic.**, cham., **Cina**, falco-p., **Iod.**, lac-eq., lach., **TARENT.**

Back

- COLDNESS, chilliness; wet cloth, as from; sacral region (2): aq-sanic., haliae-lc.

Generalities

- FOOD and drinks; fresh food, desires (4): aq-sanic., corv-c., cosm., sul-ac.

Aqua Hochstein and Birds

- RESERVED; partner, towards (2): aq-hoch., haliae-lc.
- ESTRANGED; wife, from his (13): aq-hoch., ars., bell-p., falco-p., irid., lsd, mel-alt., nat-c., phasc-c., plat., plut-n., staph., thuj.

Generalities

- SWIMMING; desires (7): *aq-hoch.*, bute-j., cyg-c., geoc-c., hema-h., lac-del., onc-t.

Aqua Taosca and Birds

- DELUSIONS, imaginations; World; he is moving in a new (7): aq-taosc., borrel., camph., corv-c., lar-ar., lsd, oplo-h.
- DREAMS; Peaceful (9): aq-taosc., coriand., *cyg-c.*, haliae-lc., hippo-k., lac-eq., *mand.*, nux-m., spig.
- SQUANDERS; money (9): aq-taosc., bac., bute-j., cinis-p., clad-r., culx-p., ind., rhodi., verat.
- FORGETFULNESS; Time, for (9): *acon.*, aq-taosc., bamb-a., cath-a., falco-p., **LACH.**, mand., merc., tax.

Generalities

- EXERCISE, exertion; desires; air, in open (7): ana-i., aq-taosc., **Fl-ac.**, kali-i., lsd, orig., teucr.
- LIGHTNING, ailments from (13): aq-taosc., bell., crot-h., cycl., dig., dpt, falco-p., lach., morph., **Nux-v.**, *phos.*, phys., sil.

Aqua Carlsbad and Birds

- MISFORTUNE; others, of, aggravates (7): aq-carl., carc., caust., **Coloc.**, corv-c., enal-c., **Tarent**.
- WEEPING, tearful mood; sympathy for others, from (14): aq-carl., bar-c., calop-s., carc., caust., cer., falco-p., irid., lyc., mand., nit-ac., puls., ros-ca-a., sep.
- DREAMS; Grief (10): all-c., alum., *amet.*, aq-carl., arist-cl., *ars.*, caust., *cyg-c.*, ros-g., stront-c.

Aqua and Fish

Vital Sensation shared = Flow

- Flow: fluid movement, momentum forwards.
- Opposite of flow = blockage, stasis, stagnant.

In the Aqua, Flow involves no effort, it simply is, a natural part of life – it can be powerful as in a mighty river, or spectacular as in a waterfall, or the last drop of rain to run down a window.

In the fishes Flow involves muscular effort to produce momentum forwards – it can also be spectacular like salmon leaping up a water fall or flying fish leaping in unison.

Vital Sensation shared = Bubble
Fish have the Vital Sensation of Bubble – as if in a bubble, yet it is different from Aqua. In the fish remedies there is a wish to escape into their bubble, their own world – a calm and pleasant place.

In Aqua they are stuck in a bubble, and/or the bubble is also stuck like a bubble in glass – there is a sense of isolation/separation about the bubble.

In Aqua there is also the physical sensation of a bubble stuck – like wind that can't be burped up, or a stream of bubbles.

Desire to Beget Children and be a Parent

This theme is especially strong in Aqua Destillata, Aqua Taosca and Oncorhyncus tshawytscha, Sockeye Salmon.

- PREGNANT, desire to be (3): aq-des., brachy-s-p., onc-t.
- CHILDREN; desires to; have, to beget, to nurture (8): aq-des., aq-taosc., lim-b-c., lsd, nat-m., *onc-t.*, ox-ac., *plac.*
- CHILDLESS, ailments from being (10): aq-des., aq-taosc., aur., lac-h., lim-b-c., lsd, nat-m., *onc-t.*, ox-ac., plac.

Useful and/or Unusual Rubrics of Aqua and Fish

Salmon = onc-t, Sea Horse = hippo-k, Goldfish = caras.

Generalities

- SWIMMING; desires (7): *aq-hoch.*, bute-j., cyg-c., geoc-c., hema-h., lac-del., onc-t. = 3 Birds and snake and milk and salmon.

- DREAMS; peaceful (9): aq-taosc., coriand., *cyg-c.*, haliae-lc., hippo-k., lac-eq., *mand.*, nux-m., spig. = 2 Birds and milk and sea horse.
- SEARCHING (14): aq-sanic., arist-cl., ars., caras., cer-i., ign., **Mag-m.**, **Nat-m.**, neod-c., plb., pras., prom., stram., verat. = Lanthanides and goldfish.

Head

- ELECTRICAL hair (6): **Aq-Sanic.**, hippo-k., imp-w., med., rhus-t., *verat.*

And last, here is a rubric to reflect upon:

- DELUSIONS, imaginations: Breathing through neck (1): aq-mar.

Aqua and Energy Remedies

The ocean is bathed in sunlight and moonlight and repeatedly struck by lightning so a relationship with Sol and Luna and Electricitas is clear to me. In the same way the natural occurrence of rainbows embraces the remedy Light Spectrum. The remedy Ultraviolet light is part of sunlight and X-Ray from cosmic radiation also continuously impinge on the earth's waters.

The magnetic field of the moon causes the ocean's tides and water is subject to the Earth's magnetic field so a relationship to the magnetic remedies of Hahnemann seems clear.

Key to energy abbreviations:

- Electricity = electr.   Light Spectrum = spect.
- Moonlight = luna.   Sunlight = sol.
- Ultraviolet light = uv-lux.   X-Ray = xray.

Magnetic field remedies of Hahnemann:

- Magnetus polus arcticus = m-arct. – north pole of magnet.
- Magetus polus australis – m-aust. – south pole of magnet.
- Magnetus artificialis = m-art. and Galvanismus = galv. – both poles of a powerful iron bar magnet – m-art also contains symptoms from placing a bar magnet on the body.

Aqua Marina and Energy Remedies: Spectrum, Ultraviolet Light, Sol

Electricitas

- DREAMS; angels, of (5): aq-mar., herin., plut-n., spect., uv-lux.
- DREAMS; control; being in (3): aq-mar., lac-cpr., *sol.*

Face

- ERUPTIONS; vesicles; cheeks (6): aq-mar., buni-o., electr., **Euph.**, syc-co., valer.

Other Aqua and Energy Remedies

- GENEROUS, too (11): aq-taosc., bos-s., bros-g., cere-b., electr., nat-m., nux-v., op., staph., sulph., thuj.
- DREAMS; desert, of (5): aq-des., herin., maia-l., *sil.*, uv-lux.
- DREAMS; cellars, vaults, crypts (6): aq-taosc., bov., caras., ilx-p., musca-d., uv-lux.

Vision

- VARIEGATED colours; sparks (2): aq-vichy-g., *galv.*

Respiration

- SNORING; expiration; sleep, in (2): *aq-carl.*, m-aust.

Extremities

- CRACKS, fissures; bleeding; hands (5): *alum.*, *aq-sanic.*, rad-br., rhus-v., x-ray

Aqua and Plants

In the Aqua the sensitivity and vulnerability is both emotional and cognitive. In the Asteraceae the sensitivity and vulnerability is to emotional wounding and in the physical body to wounding injury – cognitive function tends to remain intact except in the case of severe head/brain trauma.

There is a concordance of rubrics at the physical level and in clinical disorders – some examples are given below – many others in Chapter 10 Aqua and Clinical Applications.

Example rubrics of an Aqua with: Chrysanthemum leucanthemum, Chamomilla, Cina, Carduus benedictus, Lappa arcticum, Taraxacum officinale, Gnaphalium polycephalum, Arnica montana, Carduus marianus, Senecio aureus, Solidago virgaurea, and Echinacea angustifolia.

Aqua Sanicula and Asteraceae

- SADNESS; oppression of chest, after (2): aq-sanic., chrysan.
- CAPRICIOUSNESS; children, in (10): aq-sanic., **CHAM.**, **CINA**, **Nux-v.**, op., plac., **Puls.**, rheum, sac-alb., staph.

Generalities

- FOOD and drinks; ham; desires; fat (6): **Aq-Sanic.**, calc-p., **Carc.**, **Card-b.**, **Mez.,Tub.**

Female

- PROLAPSE; uterus; standing; aggravates (4): aq-sanic., **Lappa**, nit-ac., **Sep.**

Head

- PERSPIRATION; sleep; falling asleep, on (5): aq-sanic., *graph.*, sep., **Sil.**, **Tarax.**

Extremities

- PAIN; drawing; lower limbs; nerves, along (12): aq-sanic., cere-b., **Coff.**, dros., gels., **Gnaph.**, hyper., lac-d., **Plb.**, puls-n., staph., **Xan.**

Other Aqua and Asteraceae

Remedies: Aqua Bartfelder, Aqua Hochstein, Aqua Teplitz, Aqua Carlsbad and Aqua Hall in rubrics containing one or more asteraceae.

- ANXIETY; coffee; aggravates (5): aq-bart., **CHAM.**, *ign.*, **Nux-v.**, stram.
- GRIEF; financial loss, from (8): *aq-hoch.*, **Arn.**, ars., **Aur.**, mangi., **Mez.**, pras-o., **Psor.**

Male

- BLUE; penis (5): aq-tep., **Arn.**, ars., merc-cy., sulph.

Nose

- EPISTAXIS, haemorrhage; habitual (6): *aq-carl.*, **Card-m.**, nat-n., plb., sil., sulph.

Chest

- PAIN; burning, smarting; mammae; nipples; left (6): aq-hall, sac-l., **Senec.**, **SIL.**, spira., zinc.

Kidneys

- PAIN; extending; back, to (9): aids, aq-hoch., **BERB.**, chol., equis., graph., lac-d., **Solid.**, thymol.

Throat

- BLACK (7): aq-hoch., bism., carb-v., **Echi.**, merc-c., merc-d., merc-s.

References

1 Tumminello P. *Twelve Jewels*. Haarlem: Emryss, 1995.
2 Scholten, J. *Secret Lanthanides*. Utrecht: Stichting Alonis, 2005. pp. 46–62.

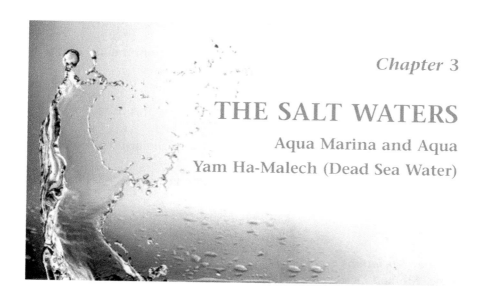

Chapter 3

THE SALT WATERS
Aqua Marina and Aqua Yam Ha-Malech (Dead Sea Water)

AQUA MARINA

Source

Water in the oceans.

History

The water in the oceans is 4 billion years old and circulates fully every 1,000 years – depths to surface, one ocean to another ocean.[1]

Content

Sodium chloride and magnesium chloride are the two major salts in sea water. Sea water contains all the soluble elements and mineral salts of the seabed and of the land it has eroded through waves and tides and had carried to it from rivers, the melting polar icecaps, rainwater, river waters and the waters of the hot and cold springs, yet like everything else, it is more than a sum of its parts.

Proving

The proving by P Sankaran[2] using sea water taken from the Bay of Biscay at a depth of 100 fathoms was published in 1963.

The proving is similar to Natrum muriaticum, but:

- Aqua Marina tans well and is not aggravated from sunshine or bright sunlight.
- Sea: there is a strong reaction – love it and ameliorated by it or aggravated by the sea.
- Salt and sea salt: strong desire or averse or aggravation.

Rubrics

Themes, Sensations and Keywords
Time, Mother, Observed and Spied Upon, Sea, Isolation, Anxiety, Fear, Angels.

Time

- Sensation as if able to look at everything from dawn of time up until today.
- Sensation as if occurrences long past were only seconds apart.
- Time past – dwells on time past – yet with less self pity and less often than Nat-m.

- DELUSIONS, imaginations; eternity; can see, of time (1): aq-mar.
- DREAMS; time; vast amounts of (1): aq-mar.
- DREAMS; time (11): acan-pl., aq-mar., bamb-a., c-di-o., cyg-b., helod-c., lsd, *onc-t.*, rhus-g., sang., telo-s.
- TIME; timelessness (14): aq-mar., ara-m., brachy-s-p., cann-i., clad-r., cyg-c., lac-lox-a., lap-c-b., *lsd*, mobil-ph., neon, onc-t., spect., tax.

Mother

- Lack of unconditional love from mother.
- Just not accepted by their mother – not acceptable as a person.
- Insignificant and overlooked by mother.

Observed and Spied Upon

- As if others are watching him – real people or disembodied beings.
- Fears that his sexual deeds and private functions are being observed.
- Unable to pass urine in front of others – toilet training – excess parental attention.

- DREAMS; spied on, of being (2): aq-mar., neon
- DELUSIONS, imaginations; Spied on, he is (5): aq-mar., bos-s., lach., med., posit.
- FEAR; looked at, when (10): aq-mar., *ars.*, bar-c., calc., germ., med., meli., ratt-n., rhus-t., tub.
- FEAR; observed, of her condition being (30): aq-mar., aq-taosc., atro., bamb-a., bar-s., beryl., **CALC.**, cer., cer-c., chel., choc., **Cimic.**, *eryth.* terb-o.
- DREAMS; nakedness, about; go home naked, can only (1): aq-mar.

Sea

- Sea of emotion ever changing – light and darkness, ever-shifting moods.
- Origins of life and evolution.
- Sensation of floating.

Isolation

- Feel alone and forgotten and abandoned.
- Lost to myself – I don't belong – not able to come back to myself.
- Insignificant and overlooked by others – as if just not seen by others – can even feel invisible.
- Reluctant to interact with others – lonely and alone.
- Aggravated in company and anxiety from public speaking.

Anxiety

- Ameliorated by: cold drinks and especially ice cold drinks, open air, walking, walking fast, walking outdoors, horse-riding, company, perspiration and wind on head.

Fears

- To go to sleep lest something should happen.
- Insanity and death.

Angels

- DREAMS; angels, of; waiting for (1): aq-mar.
- DREAMS; angels, of (5): aq-mar., herin., plut-n., spect., uv-lux.

Sensitivity and vulnerability: emotional and cognitive – loss of resilience – overwhelm

- DREAMS; control; being in (3): aq-mar., lac-cpr., *sol.*
- DREAMS; control; out of (4): aq-mar., bung-f., lam-cy., salx-f.

- SELFLESSNESS (9): anh., aq-mar., arn., iod., lant-o., nat-c., puls., rhus-t., staph.
- SELF-SUFFICIENT (12): aq-mar., calc., des-ac., erb-s., ferr-ma., gado., gins., mag-c., neod-o., neod-p., terb-s., ulm-c.
- SELF-SATISFIED (10): *aq-carl.*, aq-mar., bos-s., culx-p., fl-ac., gado., gado-n., gado-o., phasc-c., posit.

ANXIETY; ameliorated by:

- Wind on head (1): aq-mar.
- Motion; fast (2): aq-mar., saroth.
- Drinks, cold; ice cold (2): agar-em., aq-mar.
- Drinks, cold (4): **Acon.**, **Agar-em.**, aq-mar., sulph.
- Perspiration (4): agar., aq-mar., calc., camph.
- Talking; (2): aq-mar., cyg-c.
- Company (6): aq-mar., cyg-c., hura, *plac.*, rat., thul-c.

- FEAR; sleep; go to, to; lest; something should happen (2): aq-mar., sabal.

- DESPAIR; recovery, of; grief, after (1): aq-mar.
- GRIEF; pain in body, with (1): aq-mar.
- GRIEF; resigned (4): aq-mar., clem., erb., erb-o.
- GRIEF; prolonged (11): aq-mar., carc., **Caust.**, **Gels.**, **IGN.**, **Kali-br.**, **Lach.**, **Nat-m.**, **Ph-ac.**, phos., thul-m.

- SADNESS; family, for his (6): apei-s., aq-mar., ars., hep., phos., rhus-t.
- SADNESS; others, for (10): apei-s., aq-mar., ars., cocc., **Dros.**, hep., neod-c., phos., rhus-t., sulph.

- RESERVED; displeasure (6): aq-mar., **Aur.**, **Ign.**, **Ip.**, **Nat-m.**, **Staph.**

- TATTOOS, desires (1): aq-mar.
- DRESS, dresses; indecently (8): aq-mar., ephe., *hell.*, herin., **Hyos.**, salx-f., sec., **Stram.**
- EAT, eating; more than she should (11): abies-c., aq-mar., **Ars.**, bacch-a., carc., eug., helod-c., lac-del., merc-v., onc-t., thul.

DELUSIONS, imaginations:

- Divided; two parts, into; light and dark (1): aq-mar.
- Breathing through neck (1): aq-mar.
- Invisible, he is (9): aq-mar., argo., brass., **Cath-a.**, clad-r., erb., holm-c., latex, posit.
- Legs; cut off, are (8): aq-mar., bapt., **Bar-c.**, corv-c., halo., lsd, **Stram.**, tarent.

- HURRY, haste; time to arrive, for the appointed (10): aids, alum-s., aq-mar., **ARG-N.**, arist-cl., carc., culx-p., cupr., onc-t., ulm-c.

- DREAMS; romantic (12): *am-c.*, aq-mar., blatta, bung-f., coco-n., junc., **Kali-c.**, lam-cy., lap-be-e., lsd, *ros-ca-a.*, tax-br.
- DREAMS; remorse, of (22): aether, androc., aq-mar., aq-sanic., arn., ars., bros-g., caul., cocc., elaps, fl-ac., *helod-c.*, hyper., lach., led., lim-b-c., med., mobil-ph., nat-c., nat-m., plut-n., ros-g.

Suppression of emotions – Sublimation of libido

- Persistent and intruding and tormenting sexual thoughts.
- Remorse and guilt.
- Seeks salvation through prayer and the Sacraments.
- Would like to act on sexual thoughts but not able to.
- Would like to have sex but feels too weak.
- Fear of penetration.
- Impotence, incomplete erections.
- Sleepiness after masturbation.

- DREAMS; amorous; advances, unwanted (2): aq-mar., cyg-c.
- FANCIES; lascivious; tormenting (14): aq-mar., aster., bani-c., canth., coca, con., galeoc-c., graph., med., ozone, **Staph.**, stram., syph., tarent.

Male

- EMISSIONS, pollutions, seminal; dreams; with; flying, of (1): aq-mar.

Generalities

- STRETCHING; Stretch, must; emissions, pollutions, after seminal (1): aq-mar.

Exhaustion – mind and body

- MISTAKES, making; writing, in; mixes one sentence with the other (1): aq-mar.
- PROSTRATION of mind; morning (17): allox., **Aq-mar.**, arg., berb., canth., carb-v., cinis-p., galph., ilx-p., **LACH.**, lat-h., ph-ac., **Phos.**, rans., **Ruta**, *sumb.*, syph.

Head

- HEAVINESS; evening; six pm. (2): aq-mar., choc.

Generalities

- WEAKNESS; forenoon; ten a.m.; aggravates (16): aq-mar., bor., caesal-s., calc-s., cast., cench., equis., gels., lycps., merc-d., **Mur-ac.**, **Nat-c.**, ozone, **Phos.**, phys., sulph.

Useful and/or Unusual Rubrics

Head; PAIN; headache

- Forehead: clenching teeth ameliorates (1): aq-mar.
- Forehead: air, open, ameliorates (1): aq-mar.
- Occiput; motion; ameliorates (9): **Agar.**, aq-carl., aq-mar., arg., brass., euph., pip-m., **Rhus-t.**, stann.
- Sour food, after (14): **Ant-c.**, aq-mar., ars., **Bell.**, caust., ferr., ferr-p-h., lat-m., mag-p., *mand.*, morph., nat-p., **Sel.**, sulph.
- CONGESTION, hyperaemia; air, open; ameliorates (15): **APIS**, aq-mar., **Ars.**, bry., calc-s., *camph.*, caust., **Coc-c.**, ferr-i., gink., grat., hell., mag-m., mosch., *nat-c.*

Eyes

- BATHING, washing; ameliorates; sea-water, in (1): aq-mar.
- INFLAMMATION; cornea, keratitis; bath, cold, ameliorates (2): aq-mar., **Syph.**
- PAIN; burning, smarting, biting; bathing, washing; ameliorates; cold (12): **Apis**, aq-mar., ars., **Aur.**, boerh., nicc., phos., **Puls.**, **Sep.**, stront-c., tama., thuj.

Face

- ERUPTIONS; vesicles; cheeks (6): aq-mar., buni-o., electr., **Euph.**, syc-co., valer.
- PAIN; bathing, washing; aggravates (9): *am-c.*, aq-mar., calc., cench., coff., con., mag-p., neon, sil.
- WASHING; aggravates (25): **Aesc.**, **Am-c.**, aq-mar., bell., bufo, calc., camph., cench., coff., con., euph., glon., graph., **Kali-c.**, mag-p., naja, neon, nux-v., phos., phyt., sil., stann., **Sulph.**, **Thuj.**, thyr.

Nose

- INFLAMMATION; convulsive, spasmodic (2): aq-mar., cic.

Mouth

- PAIN; Palate: Morning; waking, on (2): adam., aq-mar.
- PAIN; Palate: Waking, on (6): adam., aq-mar., *bov.*, *ign.*, kali-bi., nat-c.
- PAIN; Palate: Drinks; cold, ameliorate (3): aq-mar., carc., cypr.
- PAIN; Palate; Swallowing; ameliorates (2): aq-mar., ruta.

Taste

- RUSTY; rusty, throat (2): aq-mar., tub.
- RUSTY (3): aq-mar., hydrog., tub.

Throat

- PAIN; tonsils; night (4): aq-mar., ham., ust., zinc.
- PAIN; stitching; splinters, as from; fishbone, as from (13): **Alum.**, aq-mar., **Arg-n.**, calc-s., **Carb-v.**, cinis-p., **Hep.**, **Kali-c.**, nept., **Nit-ac.**, *petr.*, phys., sac-l.
- PAIN; stitching; bone had lodged in it, as if a (19): **Alum.**, aq-mar., **Arg-n.**, **Bell.**, calc-caust., calc-s., **Carb-v.**, carbn-s., cinis-p., **Hep.**, ign., **KALI-C.**, nept., nept-m., **Nit-ac.**, phys., sac-l., **Sil.**, teucr-s.

Stomach

- APPETITE; ravenous, canine, excessive; alternating with; contentment, total (1): aq-mar.
- APPETITE; increased, hunger in general; forenoon; eleven thirty a.m., after eating (1): aq-mar.
- PAIN; bathing, washing, warm, ameliorates (2): aq-mar., salx-f.
- PAIN; Applications; warm; ameliorate (18): aq-mar., ars., atista, borrel., bry., chel., excr-can., gaul., hydr-ac., *irid.*, kali-ar., kola., lac-del., **MAG-P.**, nux-m., **Nux-v.**, salx-f., **Sil.**

Abdomen

- PAIN; rest; ameliorates (16): aq-mar., bry., *cassi-s.*, gink., grat., **Ip.**, kali-c., m-arct., *m-aust.*, nat-s., nux-m., **Nux-v.**, ox-ac., puls., *rhus-t.*, vib.
- PAIN; afternoon; aggravates; two pm. (16): aq-mar., cedr., chin-s., corn., dios., dirc., laur., lyc., mag-c., plb., ptel., rhus-t., sep., tarax., valer., verat-v.

Rectum

- CONSTIPATION; seashore, at (4): *aq-mar.*, lyc., **Mag-m.**, **Nat-m.**
- DIARRHOEA; seashore, at (6): aq-mar., **Ars.**, bry., corv-c., **Syph.**, vip.
- CONSTIPATION; home, when away from (16): **Alum.**, ambr., aq-mar., **Germ.**, **Ign.**, **Lyc.**, **M-arct.**, mag-acet., med., nat-m., **Nux-v.**, **Op.**, **PLAT.**, **Sep.**, sil., sile-c.

Bladder

- INFLAMMATION, cystitis; recurrent (16): apei-s., aq-mar., asaf., cand-a., caps., dysp-s., foll., lyc., med., morg., mut., psor., puls., sep., staph., tub.

Male

- PAIN; pushed out, as if, glans (1): aq-mar.

Female

- PAIN; uterus; squatting ameliorates (1): aq-mar.

Respiration

- DEEP; enjoyable (1): aq-mar.

Expectoration

- TASTE; rusty (1): aq-mar.

Chest

- PAIN; warmth; ameliorates (16): aq-mar., **Ars.**, *bar-c.*, caust., chel., *cimic.*, gink., harp., hep., **PHOS.**, rhus-t., rumx., sel., spong., sulph., tarent.

Back

- PAIN; Dorsal region; scapulae; angles; inferior, lower; breathing (6): alumn., aq-mar., chel., clem., cupr-ar., kali-n.
- PAIN; Rheumatic; spine, vertebrae (8): abrot., ant-s., aq-mar., cimic., euph-pu., lac-c., morg., puls.

Extremities

- ERUPTIONS; eczema; hands; palms (11) : anag., aq-mar., *aq-skook.*, asim., morg., prim-v., rad-br., **Ran-b.**, **Sulph.**, thul-o., **Vario.**

Skin

- COLDNESS; waking, on (1): aq-mar.
- CICATRICES; dark, become (2): aq-mar., sil.
- CICATRICES; itching (13): *alum.*, aq-mar., aspart., calc-f., **Fl-ac.**, **Graph.**, **Iod.**, *junc.*, **Led.**, naja, ozone, sil., tyto-a.
- ITCHING; climacteric period, in (7): aq-mar., **Arg-n.**, calad., **Canth.**, lat-m., **Murx.**, sulph.

Generalities

- BATHING, washing; ameliorates; sea, in (5): aq-mar., chir-f., hema-h., kali-i., **Med.**
- WIND; desire to be in (7): androc., aq-mar., caul., herin., hydrog., *irid.*, **Tub.**
- FOOD and drinks; honey; desires (7): aq-mar., lat-h., nat-c., nat-glut., por-m., **SABAD.**, verat.
- MONONUCLEOSIS, after effects of (11): ail., aq-mar., aq-hoch., bar-c., bar-m., calen., carc., crot-c., foll., gali., *thuj.*
- CONVULSIONS, spasms; cold; taking (15): acon., aq-mar., bell., **Caust.**, cham., chin., cic., indg., **Ip.**, lach., **Mosch.**, **Nux-v.**, sil., thuj., **Thyr.**
- CONVULSIONS, spasms; puberty, in (13): aq-mar., bufo, **Calc.**, caul., **Caust.**, cimic., cupr., hypoth., lach., nat-m., puls., zinc., zinc-val.

CASE 3.1 Psoriasis

Context

December 2003 – a 49-year-old lady with long fair hair and blue eyes attends for the first time for homeopathic treatment of severe psoriasis. She is wearing a black leather coat and trousers with a magenta blouse and scarf. She is attractive and has a powerful presence. As the case unfolds it will be seen that she has a high vitality and remarkable resilience.

Consultation 17th December 2003

I stopped work in Personnel in March. My husband has a high stress job and we had no time together. I have 3 children – twin girls and a son and have been married for 25 years.

My psoriasis began when I was 16 with the stress before exams: worse before the final school exams and college exams and better after I got married. I've had many years of steroid creams. I've never been any good with antibiotics – I feel unwell and faint and dizzy while taking them and afterwards.

Observation retrospective – *abnormal bowel flora likely – consider a bowel nosode to begin treatment.*

The psoriasis and my joints flared up badly when I was 38 – it was awful. I would wake through the night and not be able to move my fingers – they were jammed in a flexed position. I was so bad – it was terrible – I could hardly walk. I was diagnosed with psoriatic arthritis and prescribed prednisolone, but it just got steadily worse even with a lot of prednisolone. I was in despair so went for homeopathic treatment, which did help the joints to settle and I felt much better in myself and I managed to wean myself off prednisolone BUT the psoriasis stayed terrible for a whole year. I was referred to the hospital and had PUVA and lots of creams and slowly it settled down. It was bad but I could live with it.

My psoriasis has been terrible again for a whole year. The hospital prescribed cyclosporine which made me very ill with high blood pressure and raised cholesterol. It did begin to ease the psoriasis so I persevered for a while but became so ill I had to stop. Then, when I restarted it I was even worse, so I've finally stopped cyclosporine 2 weeks ago.

My psoriasis is now everywhere: dark red big patches with lots of big loose scales, **and it's so hot. I'm too hot all the time in myself as well as the skin**. My husband says I'm like a hot water bottle. I'm worse if a get hot in a hot room or from too many clothes: it feels as if it is stinging and my skin swells up in the heat. It's a bit better abroad on holiday in the sun **and much better from swimming in the sea**.

I had blood in my urine 8 years ago and cystoscopy and IVP were OK but I passed blood in my urine again last week.

Advised must not ignore blood in urine – to attend GP for repeat investigations.

My skin feels as if someone is pin-pricking me all over but worst on the left side and on my arms and now I have a pinprick rash. *Observation: she makes a wry smile*

The psoriasis goes dark red and purple as if it is almost gangrenous. At its worst it is bright red like scarlet and the itch is extreme. I could go crazy, like insane crazy, and get so angry and feel so sorry for myself. I almost crashed my car from scratching. I get so loquacious and speed-talk and drive my husband to distraction.

My skin is better in a lukewarm bath with gentle scratching while in the bath. After the bath it's much worse. Yes, I scratch while asleep and scratch till I draw blood while asleep and while awake. I was bathing in the sea in Turkey 2 years ago and felt an awful sudden sting – I'd been bitten by a doctor fish and it kept on biting me till I got out of the water and afterwards my psoriasis got better for a while.

Before exams I got anxious and had trouble remembering anything I'd read or studied – I couldn't remember any of it the next day but would remember it a week later. When well, if I learn something and it's in my brain, then it's in forever. Also I was worried that I would go blank during the exam and do less well than it was thought I would.

My mother died aged 80 of her heart and diverticulitis. My father died aged 76 – when he was 60 he got psoriasis and psoriatic arthritis.

Observation: tears appear in her eyes.

He was nice, quiet and clever and loving – I could always talk to him – we were very close. No, I didn't cry at his funeral – I was being strong for Mum.

My mother was very highly strung and had panic attacks. She never worked, she was old-fashioned and demanding. Her love was smothering and I rebelled against it.

My older brother died at 18 months old from pneumonia – he died before I was born.

I was born in the ambulance as it arrived at the hospital – my father always said that I was impatient. I have twin daughters – they were born 9 weeks early but I was confident they would both survive and they did.

There is young heart trouble in the family – my maternal grandmother died at 38 and 2 of my mother's brothers died in their 30s from heart attacks

I always feel too warm – the house is like a fridge – my husband complains it is so cold but I can't stand the central heating on.

I'm much better from sea bathing . . . my energy is 80/100 but I get very tired in the evening and can't wait to get to bed and then I don't go to sleep so I read. *When I wake in the night I'm boiling hot.* I never seem to get thirsty. My menses stopped 2 years ago and were erratic for 2 years before that. When I had periods my concentration was dreadful just before the bleeding started and better as soon as the bleeding started. The night before the bleeding starts I just feel so awful in myself and as soon as the bleeding starts I feel better.

I get a rash from red wine and loose bowels from cream and feel awful with synthetic food colours.

Direct question about her temper

I go deathly quiet before and then I explode. My temper was terrible when my daughters were 14 and 15 – I got so angry I could have killed them. When I got like that the girls would just look at me and run upstairs and once I followed them and threw everything they had onto the floor. When I go deathly angry even the dog runs away and the look frightens other people too. When I lose my temper it is awful.

Direct question about snakes

I am completely terrified of snakes – I can't even watch snakes on TV and I even find it very hard to look at a picture of a snake and it bothers me to walk through long grass in case there is a snake hiding in the grass which would bite me. No, I don't like tight clothes around my neck – I feel I will choke.

Analysis

I am sure she needs a snake and decide on Lachesis so really do not think of any further case analysis during case taking or before prescribing:

Generalities; MENSES; ameliorates; beginning of (24): all-s., alum., **Aster.**, cycl., cypra-e., glyc., hydrog., **Kali-i.**, kali-p., **Lach.**, *lap-a.*, m-aust., macrin., mag-m., mag-p., **Meli.**, *plb.*, salx-f., sapin., ser-ang., stann., verat., vib., **ZINC.**

Powerful, resilient woman with frightening violent anger and rage. Fear of snakes.

Skin pathology and symptoms worse on left side body.

Aggravation during sleep, from becoming heated, from compression around neck.

Management

Prescribed Lachesis mutans 30C 30ml drops – 2 drops in water as single dose and review response in 4 weeks – advised she may have an aggravation as she is such a vigorous strong woman, to use her usual creams more often if she does and Calendula cream 5% where skin cracks or oozes or bleeds.

Telephone Consultation 23rd December 2003

I took the dose in the evening and went to sleep quickly and had a very deep sleep without waking till morning and I woke up feeling refreshed and well but with a flare up in my psoriasis starting already in my left leg – the itch and stinging was awful and has continued. Calendula cream helps where my skin is oozing or bleeding.

Advised to not take any more doses of Lachesis for a month and then to make an appointment with me for review. She did not return till 2016.

Consultation 6th July 2016

My psoriasis has been dreadful since I saw you and I've had such a lot of powerful treatment for it since then. I really disliked taking the treatment but I took it so that I could be well enough to raise my family and to go to work.

My husband died 4 years ago and the grief has continued and my psoriasis has been much worse since he died. My husband and I met as university students and were together our whole lives.

I've been treated with methotrexate 6 months on and then off and then cyclosporine 6 months on and then off in cycles for years. In January I was prescribed a brand new drug – otzela – which has just got its licence but only managed to take it for 6 weeks because my blood pressure shot up. The cyclosporine seemed to help better than the methotrexate.

I now also have cancer of my right kidney – a clear cell adenoma stage 1, confirmed by renal biopsy and CT scan with contrast. I coughed up blood and went for tests and the chest X ray and bronchoscopy were OK but then I passed blood once in my urine and had the tests which found the kidney cancer. The surgeon has given me 3 choices – it is 3 cm now.

- I could just leave it for a year till I feel better then have an operation.
- Have cryo-ablation which has a good success rate but might need to be repeated.
- Have my kidney taken out.

I asked the surgeon what he would do himself if he had the same cancer and he said he would opt to have the kidney removed. My husband died of lung cancer.

On examination: she has the worst psoriasis I've ever seen – awful and dreadful and bright red and hot and cracking and bleeding – various sizes of patches covering more than half her skin surface but little on her face.

The itch is just terrible – it's ridiculous and I don't know how I manage to live with it.

It's much worse from heat and if I get upset. It's much worse at night and wakes me every night at exactly 1.30.

It's much better from sea bathing and much better in a salt swimming pool.

Since my husband died I've tried to be brave for everyone else's sake and have not really been able to cry. I had awful insomnia at first and am still sometimes awake till morning after I wake up at 1.30. When nursing my husband I didn't sleep well or deeply – he had awful night sweats waking 2 or 3 times each night. Some nights I was afraid to go to sleep in case he died and I would miss it. I felt hyperaware, listening to his breathing – as if I was a new mother again. I feel as if I am about to crack.

Rubrics

Skin

- ERUPTIONS; psoriasis*

Generalities

- BATHING, washing; ameliorates; sea, in (5): aq-mar., chir-f., hema-h., kali-i., **Med.**

GRIEF; silent, pent up
Generalities; CANCEROUS affections
GRIEF; ailments from, aggravates
Skin; ERUPTIONS; psoriasis; grief, after (1): staph

The renegotiation matrix generated by MacRepertory using expert analysis setting is shown in Figure 3.1.

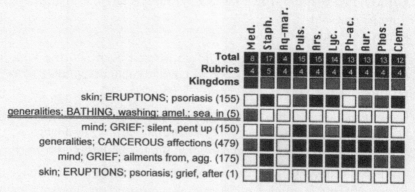

Figure 3.1 Matrix generated by MacRepertory using expert analysis setting.

Management

Staphisagria Q1 30ml, 2 drops in water once a week.
Aqua Marina 6× 30ml, 2 drops in water 6 days a week.
Repeat above cycle till a clear change and then stop (10 succussions before each dose).
Return for review in 6–8 weeks.
Begin omega 3 fish oils 3 grams daily and B multivitamins.
Nutrition: begin variety of tree nuts daily and increase variety of fruit and vegetables.
Walk quickly for 33 minutes daily no matter what the weather.

Advised to decide soon about renal surgery.

Advised that I too would personally opt for removal of kidney.

Telephone Consultation 21st July 2016

My psoriasis is 60% better already – thank you. The skin flexibility is back so I can now run up and down stairs without cracking open stiff skin. It was already obvious after a week that my psoriasis was responding to the treatment. There is now only fine scaling. BUT the itch is still the same as it was as terrible as ever and it is hard to bear.

Advised to stop Staphisagria and use creams more often even steroid creams often.

Telephone Consultation 22nd July 2016

The itch is just unbearable – it is so awful – I'm just desperate. It's driving me crazy.

I have to scratch – I must scratch – I cannot stand it if I don't scratch it and I keep scratching till I draw blood.

It's worse at night – as soon as it gets dark and worse from the heat of the bed.

Management

Psorinum Q1 30ml, 2 drops daily in water for 3 days, then 1 dose a week later, then next dose 3 weeks later.

Aqua Marina 6× – continue 2 drops daily or less often.

Consultation 22nd August 2016

The itch is coming back a bit in the last week but I'm still so much better but am confused as to what to do next with the medicines. I've got back the full flexibility of my skin and can move easily and go up and down stairs easily.

I took only one dose of Psorinum and the itch got a lot better BUT after the 1 dose the psoriasis broke out in lots of tiny patches on my arms and legs which looked different from my usual big patches, so my instinct was that I should not take any more doses.

On examination: remarkable improvement in psoriasis on body and arms – patches thin, supple and soft, much less red and much less scaly – only little scales; on legs the patches are still big and dusky red but less thick; the skin feels normal and fully flexible now on all 4 limbs.

I'm sleeping better and feel less stressed. I've had a fancy DMSA renal scan which shows a decrease in renal function: 57% in the right kidney – the 1 with the cancer – and 43% in the left kidney – so the surgeon has now advised cryotherapy first. I've had a 2nd MRI scan which shows the cancer is right in the middle of the kidney. The surgeon says that the cryotherapy can be done and repeated once if necessary. I'm hopeful that this is the right choice for me.

I took Aqua marina 6× drops twice last week – I feel it's good for me.

Management
Patient advised to restart Aqua Marina 6× drops 6 days a week.

Related Remedies

Other Aqua Remedies

Remedies: Aqua Sanicula, Aqua Skookum Chuck, Aqua Carlsbad, Aqua Teplitz, Aqua Hall.

Three rubric examples:

Eyes

• INFLAMMATION; bathing, washing; ameliorates, cold (6): **Apis**, aq-mar., aq-sanic., asar., puls., **Syph**.

Extremities

• ERUPTIONS; eczema; hands; palms (11): anag., aq-mar., *aq-skook.*, asim., morg., prim-v., rad-br., **Ran-b.**, **Sulph.**, thul-o., **Vario**.

Face

• ERUPTIONS; rash; chin (8): aids, am-c., aq-mar., aq-tep., coriand., **Dulc.**, nic-r., syph.

Invertebrate Sea Animals

Remedies: Spongia tosta, Asterias rubens, Sepia officinalis and Murex purpurea.

Five rubric examples:

• DELUSIONS, imaginations; Tormented, he is (9): **Aq-mar.**, canth., **Chin.**, Lyss., mangi., **Merc.**, soph-m., spong., zinc.

Throat

- MUCOUS, discharges; white; cotton, as (2): aq-mar., aster.
- PAIN; sore, bruised; eating; after (3): anac., aq-mar., sep.

Sleep

- SLEEPINESS; emissions, pollutions, after seminal (2): aq-mar., Sep.

Skin

- ITCHING; climacteric period, in (7): aq-mar., Arg-n., calad., Canth., lat-m., Murx., sulph.

Energy Remedies (also known as Imponderables)

Remedies: Spectrum, Ultraviolet light, Sol, Positronium and Electricitas.

Four rubric examples:

- DREAMS; angels, of (5): aq-mar., herin., plut-n., spect., uv-lux.
- DREAMS; control; being in (3): aq-mar., lac-cpr., *sol*

Face

- ERUPTIONS; vesicles; cheeks (6): aq-mar., buni-o., electr., **Euph.**, syc-co., valer.

Gemstones

Remedies: Lapis Beryllium Emerald and Adamas (Diamond).

- DREAMS; romantic (12): am-c., aq-mar., blatta, bung-f., coco-n., junc., Kali-c., lam-cy., lap-be-e., lsd, ros-ca-a., tax-br.

Mouth

- PAIN: Palate: Morning; waking, on (2): adam., aq-mar.

Lanthanides

Remedies: Lanthanum oxydatum, Holmium carbonicum, Erbium, Neodymium carbonicum, Thulium carbonicum.

Two rubric examples:

- DELUSIONS, imaginations: Invisible, he is (9): aq-mar., argo., brass., Cath-a., clad-r., erb., holm-c., latex, posit.
- DELUSIONS, imaginations: Insignificant, he is (9): aq-mar., bamb-a., cyg-c., diox., holm-c., morg., neod-c., thul-c., thul-o.

Birds

Whooper Swan (cyg-c.). Also see Luke Normand.[3]
Raven (corv-c.). Also see David Lilley.[4]

Two rubric examples:

- ANXIETY; talking; ameliorates (2): aq-mar., cyg-c.

Rectum

- DIARRHOEA; seashore, at (6): aq-mar., **Ars.**, bry., corv-c., **Syph.**, vip.

Ignatia amara and Natrum muriaticum

- RESERVED; displeasure (6): aq-mar., **Aur.**, **Ign.**, **Ip.**, **Nat-m.**, **Staph.**
- GRIEF; prolonged (11): aq-mar., carc., **Caust.**, **Gels.**, **IGN.**, **Kali-br.**, **Lach.**, **Nat-m.**, **Ph-ac.**, phos., thul-m.

Isopathic remedies – Nosodes

Remedies: Medorrhinum, Tuberculinum bovinum, Syphilinum and AIDS.

Four rubric examples:

Eyes

- INFLAMMATION; cornea, keratitis; bath, cold, ameliorates (2): aq-mar., **Syph.**
- DREAMS; hopeless (4): acan-pl., aids, aq-mar., lac-lox-a.

Generalities

- BATHING, washing; ameliorates; sea, in (5): aq-mar., chir-f., hema-h., kali-i., **Med.**
- WIND; desire to be in (7): androc., aq-mar., caul., herin., hydrog., *irid.*, **Tub.**

Isopathic remedies – Sarcodes

Remedies: Placenta humana and Thyroidinum.

Two example rubrics:

- ANXIETY; company; ameliorates (6): aq-mar., cyg-c., hura, *plac.*, rat., thul-c.

Generalities

- CONVULSIONS, spasms; cold; taking (15): acon., aq-mar., bell., **Caust.**, cham., chin., cic., indg., **Ip.**, lach., **Mosch.**, **Nux-v**, sil., thuj., **Thyr.**

AQUA YAM HA-MELACH, DEAD SEA WATER

Source

The Dead Sea is an inland lake in the River Jordan Valley with Jordan to the west and Israel to the East.

The Dead Sea is 430 metres below sea level, 304 metres deep, 50 kilometres long and 15 kilometres wide at its widest point. It is also 9 times as salty as the oceans giving it a much higher density – 1.24 kg/litre – which makes floating such a unique and lovely experience.

The water and salts and black marginal mud have been used as traditional medicine since the ancient Egyptian civilisation, mainly for skin disorders – many people now still find the bath salts soothing.

Contents[5]

Chlorides and bromides of sodium, magnesium, potassium, and calcium.

The Remedy

The sample of 100ml of water was taken 1m from the shoreline and 30cm from the water surface in the centre of the demarcated bathing area of the Dead Sea, Israel. This was evaporated and triturated by hand with lactose, then liquid potencies made in the usual way to 30 CH.

Proving

Proving by Natasha Wallace (2009) at Durban University of Technology MSc Dissertation, supervisor Dr Ingrid Couchman.[6] The proving was double blinded with 18 provers.

Rubrics

Sensitivity and vulnerability: emotional and cognitive – loss of resilience – overwhelm

Happy and energetic and euphoric and yet:

- Happiness – natural calm, relaxed happiness – crazy, silly mood – euphoria.
- Can take on the day with fury.

Alternating moods and alternating physical symptoms

- Loneliness and happiness or irritability and anxiety.
- Irritability – annoyed and agitated – frustration – impatient.
- Aggression – as if my blood is boiling – I could smash my head in – as if I could burst.

Sensation of isolation and rejection

- Intense craving for affection – needy.
- Loneliness – waves of loneliness.
- Self pity – no one understands me – go away, leave me alone.
- Questions motives and discriminates against others.

Anxiety and restlessness and fear

- Desire to escape.
- Anxiety felt in the epigastrium – sensation as if butterflies or pent up energy.
- Fears: hypochondriacal – heart attack, terminal illness, as if oxygen is not getting into my blood.

Suppression of emotions – Sublimation of libido

- Still waters run deep – fear to look too deeply at emotions.
- False front of happiness – as if a fragile mosaic front.
- Sensation of heavy burden.
- Aggravation from alcohol – loosens the suppression then more depressing.

Depression

- Deep sea of depression – bottomless.
- Waves of depression.
- Hopelessness – no light in the world.
- Death might/would be preferable.
- Uncontrolled weeping.

Exhaustion – mind and body

- As if empty – nothing left.
- Spaced out – as if floating in clouds – as if gliding – as if mind and eyes too slow to co-ordinate.
- Extremely poor concentration – unable to do any mental work.
- Procrastinating and weeping – aware work needs to be done but cannot focus brain or dry eyes.

Dehydration

- Dehydration with headache.
- Dehydration from vomiting and/or diarrhoea.
- Dryness of eyes and mouth and skin.

- Constipation with black stools.

⚠ **This symptom, even one episode, requires referral for investigation by colonoscopy, as black stools imply bleeding from the gastrointestinal tract.**

Generalities

- **Dehydration** – more than might be expected from the amount of fluid lost.
- Sensation of dryness or actual dryness of mucous membranes – eyes and gastro-intestinal tract.
- Exhaustion.
- Stiffness of muscles and joints: ameliorated by: applied heat, pressure, exercise.
- Desires: salt, cheese, coffee and alcohol.
- Averse sweets.
- Aggravation from: bright light and noise.

References

1 Carrillo J. *How old is the ocean?* Saltwater Science, Suitable 2013. Available online at: https://tinyurl.com/cx8d5hdd (Accessed 13th July 2021.)
2 Sankaran P. *British Homeopathic Journal*, 1963; 52(02): 126–132.
3 Normand L. *Animalia. A practitioner's guide to the Homeopathic Themes of 6 Animal families*. Glasgow: Saltire Books, 2021. pp. 128–131.
4 Lilley D. *The Raven. A Mythological and Comparative Study*. Glasgow: Saltire Books, 2021.

5   Ma'or Z, Henis Y, Alon Y *et al*. Antimicrobial properties of Dead Sea black mineral mud. *Int J Dermatol*. 2006, May; 45(5): 504–11.

6   Wallace N. *Homeopathic drug proving of yam ha-melach 30ch with a subsequent comparison to the materia medica of its Constituent minerals*. MSc Dissertation. Durban: Durban University of Technology, 2009. Available online at https://tinyurl.com/n3wzwx5y (Accessed 7th July 2021.)

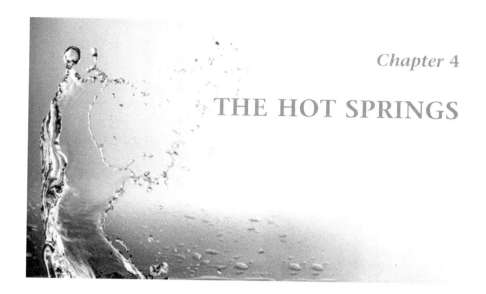

Chapter 4

THE HOT SPRINGS

The five hot springs in this chapter are Aqua Carlsbad, Aqua Cross Spring Bath, Aqua Gastein, Aqua Teplitz and Aqua Vichy Grande Grille. They are hot because of the great depth to which they flow and the length of time at that depth where they absorb radioactive elements and salts.

AQUA CARLSBAD

Source

Carlsbad Spa in the Tepla valley in the Czech Republic used the water of the 313 natural springs there for bottled water. The 2 largest and most profuse springs are hot springs used for bathing – the Sprudel and Muhlbrunnen – flowing at 39 and 41 degrees Celsius respectively which combined make the remedy *Aqua Carlsbad.*

Content

Cations in mg/l: Sodium = 1701, potassium = 79, ammonium = 0.11, calcium = 124.25, manganese = 0.09, iron = 1.34, lithium = 2.47

Anions in mg/l: Chlorine = 612.34, nitrite = 0, nitrate = 0.05, bicarbonate = 2127.13, sulphate = 1722.46, phosphate = 0.32, fluoride = 5.2[1]

Periodic table themes from:

Row 2: Carbonic acid, borax and lithium salts – carbonates and fluorides.
Row 3: Sodium and magnesium and aluminium salts – chlorides, sulphates, phosphates and silicates.
Row 4: Ferrous and manganese salts: carbonates, sulphates, phosphates, fluoride and oxides.
Row 5: Rubidium and Strontium as Iodides and bromides.
Row 6: Caesium salts.

Proving

No proving in potency – symptoms from: drinking the water and from cured cases and from symptoms from those taking Glauber's salts made by evaporation of a mixture of the waters.

Rubrics

Sensitivity and vulnerability: emotional and cognitive

- MIRTH, hilarity, liveliness; morning; waking, on (2): aq-carl., chin.
- MIRTH, hilarity, liveliness; morning (8): aq-carl., chin., con., **Fl-ac.**, graph., kola., mag-m., sulph.
- EXCITEMENT, excitable; morning; rising, on (3): *aloe*, aq-carl., iber.

- PAIN; aggravates; emotional, of others (4): aq-carl., dysp-n., erb., lim-b-c.
- MISFORTUNE; others, of, aggravates (7): aq-carl., carc., caust., **Coloc.**, corv-c., enal-c., **Tarent.**

- ANXIETY; Heart region; evening; lying down, after (3): anag., aq-carl., cench.
- ANXIETY; Heart region; evening (7): anag., aq-carl., bell., brom., cench., hydrog., **Puls.**
- ANXIETY; Constriction, with; chest, of; convulsive, spasmodic; room, aggravates in, amelioration in open air (1): aq-carl.
- ANXIETY; Constriction, with; chest, of; convulsive, spasmodic (2): aq-carl., **Cupr.**
- ANXIETY; House or room; aggravates; closed (5): aq-carl., carc., elaps, hist., sulph.

- ANXIETY; Lying; down, on, aggravates (15) and Household matters, about (16)

Heart and circulation

- APPREHENSION, region of heart (12): ant-t., aq-carl., **Aur.**, both-a., *leon.*, mand., mel-alt., meny., mez., plat., plb., **Rhus-t.**

Dreams

- Love; disappointed (1): aq-carl.
- Home; get home, trying unsuccessfully to (1): aq-carl.
- Distorting everything (3): aq-carl., **Graph.**, lac-del.
- Turtles, tortoises (3): aq-carl., germ., lac-lox-a.
- Connected; waking, after frequent (1): aq-carl.
- Grief (10): all-c., alum., *amet.*, aq-carl., arist-cl., *ars.*, caust., *cyg-c.*, ros-g., stront-c.

Loss of resilience

- SADNESS; fullness, with; stomach, in (1): aq-carl.
- SADNESS; Air, open; ameliorates (18): acon., alco., aml-n., aq-carl., arg-n., arist-cl., cann-i., cist., coff., hippo-k., irid., **Kali-c.**, laur., nat-m., **PLAT.**, **PULS.**, **Rhus-t.**, tarent.
- WEEPING, tearful mood; sympathy for others, from (14): aq-carl., bar-c., calop-s., carc., caust., cer., falco-p., irid., lyc., mand., nit-ac., puls., ros-ca-a., sep.
- SELF-SATISFIED (10): *aq-carl.*, aq-mar., bos-s., culx-p., fl-ac., gado., gado-n., gado-o., phasc-c., posit.
- MOROSE, sulky; morning; rising, on (7): aq-calc-caust., **Aq-Carl.**, canth., cham., coff., gamb., gink.
- ANGER; heat, with flushes of (7): *aq-carl.*, cham., neod-br., nux-v., *petr.*, **Phos.**, tax.
- IRRITABILITY; morning; rising, on and after (18): **Aq-Carl.**, arg-n., bry., calc., canth., carc., caul., cere-b., cham., coff., flag-l., hep., iber., mag-m., manc., nat-s., phos., sulph.

Overwhelm

- BESIDE oneself, being; trifles, about (4): **Aq-Carl.**, dros., kres., thuj.
- ANGUISH; menses; before; stretching, with (1): aq-carl.
- ANGUISH; menses; before (5): aq-carl., cocc., **Graph.**, **Murx.**, stann.

Generalities

- STRETCHING; stretch, must; anguish, during (2): androc., aq-carl.

Suppression of emotions – Sublimation of libido

- DREAMS; lewd, lascivious, voluptuous; emissions, pollutions, with seminal; old people, in (1): aq-carl.

Abdomen

- MURMURING, muttering (2): *aq-carl.*, sabad.

Back

- FORMICATION, crawling; extending; downward (1): aq-carl.
- FORMICATION, crawling; dorsal region; scapulae; between (6): anac., aq-carl., c-di-o., *laur.*, m-arct., *viol-t.*

Face

- FORMICATION, crawling; cheeks (16): acon., *agn.*, *aq-carl.*, Arn., bar-c., brom., carc., cench., elaps, *euon.*, Euph., *grat.*, *helo.*, lar-ar., *nux-v.*, uv-lux.

Abdomen

- BAND around; Ring around, like a, deep respiration aggravates (1): **Aq-Carl.**

Back

- TWITCHING; coccyx (7): alum., aq-carl., carb-an., caust., chin., **Cic.**, rhus-t.
- TWITCHING; coccyx; extending; bladder, to (2): aq-carl., carb-an.
- TWITCHING; coccyx; extending; prepuce, to (1): aq-carl.

- ERECTIONS, troublesome; Causeless (6); Stool; during (6)

- YAWNING
- Forenoon; nine am. (2); Drinking aggravates (1); Hiccough, in (7); Menses; before (4); Sitting, while (8); Stretching, with

Desire to Beget Children and Be a Parent

Abdomen

- MOVEMENTS; foetus, as of; first movement (1): aq-carl.
- MOVEMENTS; foetus, as of (16): aq-carl., bacch-a., cinis-p., con., conv., **Croc.**, latex, *leon.*, **Nat-c.**, sabin., sals-t., stann., **Sulph.**, tarent., **Ther.**, **THUJ.**

- LOVE; children, for (24): acet-ac., aq-carl., aq-taosc., **Ars.**, chlor., excr-can., ferr-i., gins., **Hep.**, joan., kali-bi., kali-m., lac-eq., lim-b-c., niob., onc-t., ox-ac., ph-ac., phos., *plac.*, plat., sep., verbe-o., *xan.*

Exhaustion – mind and body

- DISCOURAGED; menses; before (1): aq-carl.
- DISCOURAGED; domestic duties, about (1): aq-carl.
- HEEDLESS, careless; talking and writing, in (1): aq-carl.
- FORGETFULNESS; night; talking, while (1): aq-carl.
- FORGETFULNESS; night (8): aq-carl., chin., lyc., op., plat., sarr., sil., sulph.

CONFUSION of mind

- Motion; ameliorates (5): **Ant-t.**, *aq-carl.*, arg-n., ferr., ferr-p.
- Walking; ameliorates; air, in open (13): **Aq-Carl.**, bry., digin., graph., LYC., merc-i-f., merc-i-r., nat-c., par., **PULS.**, rhod., salx-f., sulph.

Unique rubrics

- Eyes; LACHRYMATION; Sewing, from (1): **Aq-Carl.**
- Vision; SPARKS; Streaks in, after writing (1): **Aq-Carl.**
- Ears; TWITCHING; Eustachian tubes, boring with finger ameliorates (1): **Aq-Carl.**
- Nose; SNEEZING; Menses; suppressed, from (1): **Aq-Carl.**
- Extremities; COLDNESS; Fingers; tips; writing, after (1): **Aq-Carl.**
- Extremities; COLDNESS; Toes; sitting; after (1): **Aq-Carl.**
- Kidneys; HEAVINESS; Sitting aggravates (1): **Aq-Carl.**
- Kidneys; PAIN; Ureters extending to prepuce (1); **Aq-Carl.**
- Head; SENSITIVENESS of Skull, bones; periosteum (1): *aq-carl.*
- Face; COBWEB sensation; Cheek bone, right (1): *aq-carl.*

Clinical Rubric Clusters

Heartburn and Hiccoughs ameliorated by cold drinks

Stomach

- PAIN; Burning; supper, after (1): aq-carl.
- HEARTBURN: Afternoon; riding, while (1): aq-carl.
- HEARTBURN; Diet, after disturbance of (1): aq-carl.

- ERUCTATION; Fluid; forenoon (1): **Aq-Carl.**
- ERUCTATION; Eggs; rotten, spoiled, like; evening (1): aq-carl.
- ERUCTATION; waterbrash; salty (15): aq-carl., bry., calc., **Carb-an.**, **Caust.**, euph., lyc., mag-m., merc., **Phos.**, rhus-t., sep., sul-ac., tarax., verb.

- HICCOUGH; breakfast; after (4): alum., aq-carl., **Tarent.**, **Zinc.**

- HICCOUGH; yawning; while (8): **Aml-n.**, aq-carl., card-b., caust., **Cocc.**, **Cycl.**, **Mag-c.**, nat-m.

Chest

- CONTRACTION; Cardiac orifice; dinner, after (1): aq-carl.

Headaches

PAIN, headache:

- Tearing; occiput; motion; ameliorates (1): aq-carl.
- Tearing; temples; motion; ameliorates (1): aq-carl.
- Tearing; motion; ameliorates (8): *act-sp.*, *aq-carl.*, caps., kali-i., mur-ac., **Rhod.**, **Rhus-t.**, sulph.

- Burrowing; sides (7): **Agar.**, aq-carl., bry., chin., clem., phos., rat.
- Pressing; temples; daytime (4): aq-carl., cer-p., hep., **Stann.**
- Temples; motion; ameliorates (8): aq-carl., calc., com., ferr., lil-t., merc., **Mez.**, psor.
- Occiput; motion; ameliorates (9): **Agar.**, aq-carl., aq-mar., arg., brass., euph., pip-m., **Rhus-t.**, stann.
- PULSATION; vertex; ascending stairs aggravates (2): aq-carl., ferr.
- PULSATION; ascending, on (9): alum., aq-carl., aster., **Bry.**, carl., ferr., glon., nat-p., par., **Sep.**

- SENSITIVENESS; skull, bones; periosteum (1): *aq-carl.*
- SENSITIVENESS; skull, bones (6): aq-carl., kali-bi., **Kali-hp.**, *kali-n.*, *phos.*, *squil.*

Rheumatic problems

Pain and inflammation of joints hands and feet previously frozen in frostbite

Extremities; PAIN:

- Toes; frozen, after being (3): agar., carl., phos.
- Feet; heels; frozen, formerly (4): aq-carl., phos., puls., *sabin.*
- Aching; feet; heels; frozen, formerly (1): aq-carl.
- Toes; frozen, formerly (1): aq-carl.
- Burning, smarting; toes; frozen, formerly (3): agar., aq-carl., phos.
- Burning, smarting; nettles, as from; hands; back (2): aq-carl., harp.

- Stitching; rhythmical, feet; heels (1): aq-carl.
- Stitching; rhythmical, feet (2): aq-carl., nat-m.

Back pain: lumbar and coccyx extending to groin and genitals and bladder

Back

- PAIN; lumbar region, lumbago; lassitude, with (1): *aq-carl.*,
- PAIN; lumbar region, lumbago; extending to; lower limbs; bending backward and on raising the body (1): aq-carl.,
- PAIN; lumbar region, lumbago; extending to; abdomen; pubis; inguinal region, and (2): *aq-carl.*, kreos.
- PAIN; lumbar region, lumbago; extending to: genitals (12): abrot., **Aq-Carl.**, berb., cadm., dros., erig., gran., **Kali-c.**, kreos., osm., sars., sulph.

- PAIN; extending to; bladder (4): aq-carl., bell., **BERB.**, fl-ac.
- PAIN; aching; paralytic, lumbar region (8): aq-carl., **Cocc.**, kalm., nat-m., ran-s., **Sabin.**, sel., zinc.
- PAIN; drawing; lumbar region; menses; during (6): am-m., aq-carl., calc., cham., *mag-c.*, sep.
- PAIN; pressing; lumbar region; extending to; genitals (2): *aq-carl.*, **Kali-c.**
- PAIN; stitching; lumbar region; extending; pelvis, to (1): *aq-carl.*
- PAIN; stitching; lumbar region; extending; abdomen, to; pubis and inguinal region, to (2): *aq-carl.*, kreos.

- PAIN; coccyx, coccygodynia; extending; prepuce, to (1): aq-carl.
- PAIN; coccyx, coccygodynia; extending; bladder, to (2): aq-carl., fl-ac.

- PARALYSIS; lumbar region; rising, after (1): aq-carl.
- STIFFNESS; painful; left (7): *am-m.*, *aq-carl.*, chlorpr., gink., *nit-ac.*, **Sep.**, trio.
- TENSION; lumbar region; extending to; genitals (1): *aq-carl.*
- HEAT; alternating with; chill (5): *aq-carl.*, cham., erech., merc-c., **Verat.**

Irritable bowel syndrome

Abdomen

- PAIN; coffee; ameliorates (4): aq-carl., **Cham.**, **COLOC.**, con.
- PAIN; boring; spleen region (5): aq-carl., kali-bi., *nat-m.*, nelum., seneg.

- PAIN; electric, like; hypogastrium (1): aq-carl.
- PAIN; electric, like (12): aml-n., aq-carl., **Arg-n.**, berb., carl., caust., **Coloc.**, geum, **Kreos.**, pip-n., sapin., stry., **Thal-s.**

- TENSION; dinner, after (5): aq-carl., cycl., nit-ac., plat., sulph.
- PULSATION; lying, while (5): aloe, aq-carl., aran-ix., **Coloc.**, plb.

- FULLNESS; eating; ameliorates (2): aq-carl., *rhus-t.*
- FULLNESS; afternoon (11): aq-carl., caesal-s., clem., coca, con., ferr-m., mag-c., myric., phyt., plan., plb.

- HEAVINESS as from a load or weight:
- Drinking aggravates; water (1): aq-carl.
- Drinking aggravates (3): aq-carl., **Asaf.**, sin-a.
- Menses; beginning of (1): aq-carl.
- Afternoon (7): alum., aq-carl., chin., dios., ser-ang., ter., tong.

- ROUGHNESS, scraping sensation; coffee ameliorates (1): aq-carl.
- ROUGHNESS, scraping sensation (13): aesc., **Aq-Carl.**, **Arg.**, *camph.*, dig., dros., mang-acet., nat-m., nux-v., plb., ruta, *sabad.*, sulph.

Bunion: inflamed and pain in wet weather

- INFLAMMATION; Toes; first; ball; swelling, with, bunion; weather, in damp, wet (1): aq-carl.

Useful and/or Unusual Rubrics

Generalities

- FOOD and drinks; Bread; desires; rye bread (8): anis., aq-carl., **Ars.**, ign., nat-m., plb., psor., sama-sil.

Hearing

- NOISES; writing, while (3): aq-carl., sep., zinc.

Eyes

- WEAKNESS; writing, while (4): aq-carl., bell., **NAT-M.**, **Sep.**
- TWITCHING; canthi: Inner; right (5): **Aq-Carl.**, chel., rat., stann., *sul-ac.*

Face

- HAIR sensation (12): aq-carl., bacch-a., chlol., echis-c., euphr., **Graph.**, *irid.*, laur., led., mobil-ph., sulph., **Sumb.**

Abdomen

- COLDNESS; extending; chest, to (3): aq-carl., camph., par.
- CONSTRICTION; band sensation; ring around, like a, deep respiration aggravates (1): **Aq-Carl.**
- CONTRACTION; diaphragm; respiration, on (1): aq-carl.
- CONTRACTION; diaphragm (11): aconin., aq-carl., asaf., asar., canth., cench., cypr., dros., led., mez., **Nux-v.**
- CONTRACTION; umbilical region; sitting ameliorates (1): *aq-carl.*
- CONTRACTION; umbilical region; stooping ameliorates (1): *aq-carl.*

- GURGLING; fluid, as from (11): **Aq-Carl.**, **Arum-d.**, asim., cortico., cortiso., **Croto-t.**, **Jatr.**, *ph-ac.*, *plat.*, sin-a., *sul-ac.*

Chest

- HEAVINESS; suffocated feeling, with (4): *aq-carl.*, nitro., ptel., spig.
- OPPRESSION; exertion, from (10): adren., **Am-c.**, *aq-carl.*, ars., **Aur.**, **Calc.**, **Ferr.**, nat-ar., pier-b., sulph.

Heart and circulation

- TENSION; heart, region of (5): *aq-carl.*, sec., torul., **Zinc.**, *zinc-o.*
- PAIN; pressing; region of; left (5): *aq-carl.*, chel., lyc., thuj., **Zinc.**

Larynx and trachea

- ROUGHNESS, scraping sensation (13): aesc., **Aq-Carl.**, **Arg.**, *camph.*, dig., dros., mang-acet., nat-m., nux-v., plb., ruta, *sabad.*, sulph.

Respiration

- DEEP; oppression, with; chest, of (8): *aq-carl.*, cadm., **Cann-s.**, carc., **Caust.**, *croc.*, **Plat.**, sin-a.

Kidneys

- PAIN; pressing; sitting, while (6): aq-carl., **Caust.**, pall., ruta, **Ter.**, thuj.
- PAIN; aching; region of; left (8): acon., agar., aq-carl., chin-s., croto-t., elat., equis., pall.

Extremities

- SHOCKS; knees (9): **Agar.**, aq-carl., **Arg.**, **Arn.**, m-art., **Puls.**, sul-ac., **Valer.**, verat.

Sleep

- LIGHT; midnight; about (1): aq-carl.
- LIGHT; midnight; after (4): ant-s., aq-carl., coc-c., grat.
- YAWNING; morning; breakfast, after (1): aq-carl.
- YAWNING; drinking aggravates (1): aq-carl.
- YAWNING; forenoon; nine am. (2): aq-carl., lyc.
- YAWNING; menses; before (4): am-c., aq-carl., phel., **PULS.**

Related Remedies

Aqua

Remedies: Aqua Marina, Aqua Taosca, Aqua Sanicula, Aqua Adelheid, Aqua Wiesbaden.

Head

- PAIN, headache; Occiput; motion; ameliorates (9): **Agar.**, aq-carl., aq-mar., arg., brass., euph., pip-m., **Rhus-t.**, stann.

Vision

- FLICKERING; reading, from (14): *aq-carl.*, aq-lipp., aran., arn., *bell.*, cob., **Cycl.**, hell-f., *lach.*, merc., *merl.*, onc-t., *ph-ac.*, **Seneg.**

Throat

- PAIN; sore, bruised; uvula (13): am-m., aq-carl., aq-sanic., calc., canth., caust., chlor., nat-ar., nit-ac., ptel., ruta, sabin., **Sang.**

Abdomen

- RUMBLING noise; coffee ameliorates (3): aq-adel., aq-carl., phos.

Female

- MENSES; return after having ceased, periods; climacteric period, in (7): aq-carl., aq-wies., lyss., mag-c., phos., sile-c., thea.

Post-Menopausal Bleeding requires referral to a gynaecologist for investigation, diagnosis and management. Homeopathy would be supportive treatment.

Lanthanides

Remedies: Dysprosium nitricum, Erbium, Neodymium bromatum, Gadolinium, Gadolinium nitricum, Gadolinium oxydatum, Samarium silicatum.

- PAIN; aggravates; emotional, of others (4): aq-carl., dysp-n., erb., lim-b-c.
- ANGER; heat, with flushes of (7): *aq-carl.*, cham., neod-br., nux-v., *petr.*, **Phos.**, tax.
- SELF-SATISFIED (10): *aq-carl.*, aq-mar., bos-s., culx-p., fl-ac., gado., gado-n., gado-o., phasc-c., posit.

Generalities

- FOOD and drinks; Bread; desires; rye bread (8): anis., aq-carl., **Ars.**, ign., nat-m., plb., psor., sama-sil.

Metals – Share and Compare Clinical Rubrics

Row 4: Cuprum and Zinc.
Row 5: Stannum and Cadmium and Palladium and Tellurium.

Row 6: Platinum and Aurum and Plumbum and Iridium.

One rubric example is shown for each metal.

Row 4 metals: Cuprum and Zinc

- ANXIETY; constriction, with; chest, of; convulsive, spasmodic (2): aq-carl., **Cupr.**

Heart and circulation

- TENSION; heart, region of (5): *aq-carl.*, sec., torul., **Zinc.**, *zinc-o.*

Row 5 metals: Stannum, Argentum, Cadmium, Palladium, Tellurium

Stannum

Head

- PAIN, headache; Pressing; temples; daytime (4): aq-carl., cer-p., hep., **Stann.**

Argentum

Larynx and trachea

- ROUGHNESS, scraping sensation (13): aesc., **Aq-Carl.**, **Arg.**, *camph.*, dig., dros., mang-acet., nat-m., nux-v., plb., ruta, *sabad.*, sulph.

Cadmium

Respiration

- DEEP; oppression, with; chest, of (8): *aq-carl.*, cadm., **Cann-s.**, carc., **Caust.**, *croc.*, **Plat.**, sin-a.

Palladium

Kidneys

- PAIN; pressing; sitting, while (6): aq-carl., **Caust.**, pall., ruta, **Ter.**, thuj.

Tellurium

Kidneys

- HEAVINESS (18): *absin.*, aeth., androc., **Aq-Carl.**, benz-ac., **Cimic.**, dirc., equis., **Helon.**, hydrc., **Juni-c.**, nux-v., phos., pic-ac., **Sang.**, tax., tell., **Ter.**

Row 6 metals: Aurum, Iridium, Platinum, Plumbum

Aurum

Heart and circulation

- APPREHENSION, region of heart (12): ant-t., aq-carl., **Aur.**, both-a., *leon.*, mand., mel-alt., meny., mez., plat., plb., **Rhus-t.**

Iridium

Eyes

- TWITCHING; canthi; inner (8): **Aq-Carl.**, chel., *irid.*, kali-chl., lycpr., rat., stann., sul-ac.

Platinum

Extremities

- FORMICATION, crawling: Sitting, while (11): aq-carl., bar-c., carc., **Guai.**, kali-c., mag-m., ol-an., **Plat.**, staph., teucr., zing.

Plumbum

Abdomen

- CONSTRICTION; bowels (8): *aq-carl.*, astac., chion., **Coloc.**, **Plb.**, **Spig.**, **Ter.**, **Thuj.**

Carbons – Share and Compare Clinical Rubrics

Remedies: Graphites, Carbo vegetabilis, Carbo animalis and Terebinthiniae oleum.

- ANGUISH; menses; before (5): aq-carl., cocc., **Graph.**, **Murx.**, stann.

Chest

- OPPRESSION; eructation ameliorates (9): **Am-m.**, *aq-carl.*, calc., **CARB-V.**, *grat.*, **Lach.**, *lact.*, **LYC.**, **Phos.**

Larynx and trachea

- PAIN; raw; larynx; morning (11): aq-carl., calc., **Carb-an.**, **Caust.**, cob., **Iod.**, **Rhus-t.**, **Sil.**, **Stann.**, **SULPH.**, zinc.

Abdomen

- CONSTRICTION; bowels (8): *aq-carl.*, astac., chion., **Coloc.**, **Plb.**, **Spig.**, **Ter.**, **Thuj.**

Kidneys

- PAIN; pressing; sitting, while (6): aq-carl., **Caust.**, pall., ruta, **Ter.**, thuj.

Acids – Share and Compare Clinical Rubrics

Remedies: Fluoric acid, Sulphuric acid, Nitric acid and Phosphoric acid.

- MIRTH, hilarity, liveliness; morning (8): aq-carl., chin., con., **Fl-ac.**, graph., kola., mag-m., sulph.

Eyes

- TWITCHING; canthi: inner; right (5): **Aq-Carl.**, chel., rat., stann., *sul-ac.*

Male

- FORMICATION, crawling; scrotum (18): acon., **Aq-Carl.**, *berb.*, *carb-v.*, chel., *chin.*, clem., com., *merc.*, *nit-ac.*, **Ph-ac.**, plat., rhus-v., **SEC.**, sel., *sil.*, **Staph.**, *thuj.*

Sarcodes – Share and Compare Clinical Rubrics

Remedies: Corticotrophinum, Cortisone, Adrenalinum and Atropinum Purum.

Abdomen

- GURGLING; fluid, as from (11): **Aq-Carl.**, **Arum-d.**, asim., cortico., cortiso., **Croto-t.**, **Jatr.**, *ph-ac.*, *plat.*, sin-a., *sul-ac.*

Chest

- OPPRESSION; exertion, from (10): adren., **Am-c.**, *aq-carl.*, ars., **Aur.**, **Calc.**, **Ferr.**, nat-ar., pier-b., sulph.

Sleep

- YAWNING; sitting, while (9): aq-carl., atro., bor., clem., cocc., nat-c., nicc., tarax., *viol-t.*

Physiology of standing head out of water immersion in thermal waters[2]

Cardiovascular, renal and hormonal changes in normal subjects and in those with early lead toxicity were noted after standing head out of water immersion (SHOWI) in Bath spa water and plain tap water at temperatures from 33° to 39° Celsius at immersion times of 1, 2 and 3 hours. The greatest changes occurred with immersion at 37°C (the bathing temperature in the Cross Bath was a constant 37.7°C).

Cardiovascular

Significant (p less than 0.001) rise in cardiac index and stroke volume and fall in peripheral resistance were found. The percentage rise in cardiac output rose from 34% at 35°C to 80% at 37°C.

Renal

The increase in diuresis was found to be most stable at 37°C. There was haemo-dilution with fall in haemoglobin, red cell count and plasma viscosity; increase in urine volume and increased excretion of sodium, potassiuom, calcium and lead.

Hormonal

Decrease in the secretion of anti-diuretic hormone, rennin, aldosterone and catecholamines, and increase in the secretion of atrial natriuretic peptide.

Although there were differences in results between tap water and Bath spa water these were deemed not statistically significant.

AQUA CROSS SPRING IN BATH

Source

Aqua Cross Spring in Bath remedy made by Helios Pharmacy in Kent, UK from fresh water of the Cross Spring in Bath, Somerset, England collected during routine bacteriological testing by employees of Bath City Council.

Content

A chemical analysis of the water from Bath Cross Spring reveals: total mineralisation 2295, ph 6.9, Calcium 393, Sodium 220, Magnesium 58, Potassium 18, Sulphate 1080, Chloride 325, Bicarbonate 170, Nitrate 0.35, Strontium 6.3, Iron 2.0, Barium 0.03, Boron 0.5, Silicon 19.5, Manganese 0.3, Bromine 1.8, Iodine 0.041, traces of Radon, Helium, Radium and Uranium.[3]

The chemical composition of the water shows it has chemically equilibrated with carboniferous limestone with little influence from rainfall or superficial ground water.

Proving

Proving by Dr Raymond Sevar in 2000.[4]

Rubrics

Radio-active contents of the Cross Spring – Radon, Helium, Radium and Uranium[5]

The largest contributor to the spring's radioactivity is Radon: $Radon^{222}$ 800 picocuries/l; $Helium^4$ 700 picocuries/l, $Radium^{226}$ 10.2 picocuries/l, Uranium 0.055 micrograms/l (U^{234}/U^{238} activity ratio 2.77). The radio-element contents, although greater than shallow ground water, are an insignificant hazard for public tasting of the waters.

Age of the water of the Cross Spring

Best estimates are that the water is between 3000–10,000 years old. The isotope composition and noble gas recharge temperatures of the water shows that it was recharged within the last 10,000 years. The Uranium U^{234}/U^{238} activity ratio suggests the water has resided deep in the Carboniferous limestone for 3,000 years. A geo-thermal gradient of 20°C/km indicates water circulation to a depth of 2,500 metres.

Themes, Sensations and Keywords

Sensitivity and vulnerability: emotional and cognitive – loss of resilience – overwhelm

- Intuitive premonition of suffering and pain.
- Sympathetic to others suffering and pain.
- Rage followed by severe and persistent oesophageal pain.
- Death and grief.
- Poison and nausea.
- Heaviness and exhaustion.
- Thirst with desire for still, filtered water.

Sympathetic

- Heart feeling very open for a misunderstood colleague – the feeling was well localised to the heart – lasting two days.

Rage

- Uncontrollable rage for two days with lots of tears – my husband was actually frightened of me and thought that I would divorce him.
- Rage followed by severe and persistent burning oesophageal pain.

Grief

- Overwhelming grief at the Earth's plight, a feeling of great grief for Gaia lasting two days.

Overwhelmed

- I want to be alone.
- I want to escape – it must be to a high open hill with trees – it must have trees – the desire to be alone lasted two days.
- Internal restlessness at night.

Death

- Desire for death, I really wanted to die for two days.
- I really wanted to cut my throat.

Poison and nausea

- This remedy is poison, real deep poison – the feeling lasted for five days.

Nausea

- Nausea began one minute after the first dose and persisted for 44 days.
- Nausea worse from: eating, pressure, evenings.
- Nausea ameliorated by walking.
- Nausea associated with jaundice, sour flatulence, increase in appetite even though eating aggravates, weight gain, oppression of the chest, pain in liver, a sharp pulsating stabbing pain in xiphisternum.

Burning pain in oesophagus

- Throughout whole length of my oesophagus – lasted 38 days and began as the emotional symptoms resolved.
- Linear central pain well localised to my oesophagus – upper, middle, lower or whole length.
- Ameliorated by eating – I must eat every two hours, or the pain is terrible.
- Despite eating regularly lost three kg in weight.

Thirst

- Unquenchable severe thirst.
- Desire to drink many litres of water.
- Desire for still, filtered water.
- Aversion sparkling mineral water.

Heaviness and Depth

- I felt my arm sinking down with the weight of the remedy as I hold the bottle.
- I feel as if the remedy is from deep in the earth.
- Oppressive weight in upper chest with a strong well localised feeling of heartache for five days.

- Whole body feels as if heavy.
- Left side of body feel heavier and more robust and somehow calmer than the right.

Head Pain

- Headache and band sensation – occipital and spreading forwards – congested, full and tight.
- Ameliorated by eating and fresh air.
- Aggravated by thinking and concentrating on mental work.
- Accompanied by a hot, hard and tight feeling in eyeballs and eyelids feel hot along the lid margins.
- Head pain boring inwards above left eye of sudden onset – periodicity 10 days.
- Headache with pain deep behind my eyes settling into a sharp pain in left eye.
- Headache from early morning gradually increasing to bursting in vertex and occiput aggravated by glaring light and better from a walk in the fresh open air – persisting for two days.
- Headache behind eyes – pain well localised in bones of maxillae and ethmoid plates lasted for two days.

Dreams of Water

- Going to get water for an allotment from a large pond.
- Driving a lorry with kids on snow, helping a cyclist who'd slipped on snow and then cycling on snow.
- In a room with lino on the floor, snake-like bulge under the lino, felting nails holding down lino – I thought that water under the lino would fountain out of the nail holes – what did come out of the bulge was a small creature.

Dreams

- Being taught by a great Master – he'd something hugely important to tell me, but I woke up before he could.
- Castles.

Sensations as if

- I have moved my bowels but do not feel finished and the sensation persists some time.
- Left side of body feels calmer, heavier and more robust.
- 12 noon – a woolly sensation over my forehead.
- Left corner of mouth felt as if cracked.

- My feet feel hot inside but are cold to touch.
- My feet feel swollen but are not.

Generals

- Sensation of being so cold inside that nothing would warm me up – even on warm days -persisted for five days.
- I'm so chilly that I have to wear a down-filled jacket indoors.
- Burning: pain in oesophagus and burning sensation of heat in feet at night in bed – must uncover feet.
- Desire for salt and I am usually averse.
- Desire for vinegar and I am usually averse.

Rheumatic

- Severe sharp pain in sacro-iliac joints, felt deep in the joints.
- Pain in lumbar spine radiating and extending to the back of my thighs.
- Pain – deep at the level of connective tissue.
- Sharp pain in right Achilles tendon made better by walking.

AQUA GASTEIN

Source

The hot springs of Wildbad Gasterin in Salzburg, Austria.

Content

The springs contain a natural colloidal suspension of fine pure white particles of calcium silico-fluoride = Lapis albus.

Sodium sulphate is the most abundant mineral in the spring whose contents are:

Row 2: Lithium chloride, carbonic acid.
Row 3: Sodium sulphate, magnesium carbonate, aluminium phosphate, silicic acid.
Row 4: Potassium carbonate, potassium sulphate, calcium fluoride, calcium silico-fluoride = lapis albus particles, titanic acid, ferrous carbonate, arsenic.
Row 5: Rubidium and strontium salts.
Row 6: Caesium salts.

Remedy made by trituration of the evaporated water – the remedy *Aqua Gastein* contains *Lapis albus* and all its effects and symptoms.

Rubrics

Sensitivity and vulnerability: emotional and cognitive – loss of resilience – overwhelm

- EXCITEMENT, excitable; bath, during a (1): aq-gast.
- ANXIETY; orgasm of blood, with (12): **Acon.**, aloe, **Am-m.**, aq-gast., **Bar-c.**, carb-an., chel., merl., nit-ac., plb., **Puls.**, **Sep.**

Abdomen

- UNCERTAINTY, feeling of (1): aq-gast.

Chest

- PAIN; weight of jacket, from (1): aq-gast.

Suppression of emotions – Sublimation of libido

Male

- ERECTIONS; involuntary (7): acon-c., **Anac.**, aq-gast., bell., clem., curc., tarax.

Water

- Great accumulation of water in the mouth after dinner.
- Discharge of clear water from the mouth.
- Thirst increased and drinks a lot of water.

Exhaustion – mental and physical

- Children with goitre with large appetite.
- Children with large and chronic enlarged lymph nodes in neck – aq-gast. and lap-a.
- OBESITY; Young people, in; children; fat anaemic babies with iodine appetite (1): aq-gast.

Clinical Rubric Clusters

Skin: Eruptions, Tumours and Scars

- Tumours lips.
- Boils and vesicles – painful and burning and smarting.
- Scars crack and become covered or surrounded by painful vesicles.

Face

- TUMOURS; lips; lower (3): aq-gast., lap-a., phos.
- TUMOURS; lips (10): aq-gast., ars-i., **Con.**, cupre-l., galph., kreos., lap-a., phos., sep., vinc.

Skin

- CICATRICES; cracked (4): aq-crot-h., **Graph.**, *kali-c.*
- CICATRICES; vesicles, covered or surrounded by itching (3): aq-gast., **Fl-ac.**, mag-c.
- ERUPTIONS; pimples; yellow (3): ant-c., aq-gast., crot-c.
- ERUPTIONS; pimples; subcutaneous (5): alum., alumn., aq-gast., raph., stel.

Extremities

- CALLOSITIES, horny; painful; hand, palm, right (1): aq-gast.

Heartburn and Irritable Bowel Syndrome

Water-brash and eructation – is frequent or constant and unpleasant, with loss of appetite and nausea.

Stomach

- ERUCTATIONS; morning; swallow, must (1): aq-gast.
- ERUCTATIONS; water-brash; pain, with; stomach, in (14): acet-ac., aq-gast., asaf., bism., bism-n., caps., caust., cic., graph., lyc., nux-v., petr., psor., sulph.

Abdomen

- PAIN; dragging, bearing down; Heavy, as if too (1): aq-gast.
- PAIN; dragging, bearing down; Extending; downward (8): all-s., aloe, aq-gast., **Bry.**, coc-c., lact., til., vib.
- PAIN; bowels; caecum (7): ammc., aq-gast., caust., coloc., *croto-t., gnaph.*, merc-c.

Rectum

- PAIN; stitching; left (3): aq-gast., chim., **Croc.**

Useful and/or Unusual Rubrics

Generalities

- STRENGTH; increased; walking, while (4): aq-gast., bapt., chin,, zinc.
- COLD; taking, easily; abnormally easy (6): aq-gast., merc., nit-ac., pitu-a., solid., sulph.

Head

- PAIN, headache; pressing; forehead; vertigo; after (1): aq-gast.

Hearing

- NOISES; TRUMPETS, like (3): aq-gast., *bell.*, chin-b.
- NOISES; REAL, seem (1): aq-gast.

Female

- FORMATIONS, fibrous membranous, from uterus (1): aq-gast.
- LEUCORRHEA; membranous (10): aq-gast., **Bor.**, bov., hep., hydr., kali-bi., lept., nit-ac., phyt., vib.

Chest

- PERSPIRATION; red; axillae (8): aq-gast., arn., **Carb-v.**, dulc., **LACH.**, **NUX-M.**, nux-v., thuj.

Heart and circulation

- PAIN; pressing; heart region; evening (8): aq-gast., helo., lycps., **Nat-m.**, **PULS.**, ser-ang., sulph., thuj.

Back

- COLDNESS, chilliness; creeping (9): aq-gast., bell., calc-ar., equis., lac-d., med., merc-c., nux-m., sil.

Extremities

- CONSTRICTION; band sensation; iron; upper limbs (2): aq-gast., cact.
- PAIN; stitching; splinters, as from; fingers; fourth, ring, first phalanx (1): aq-gast.

Aqua Gastein: Compare and Related Remedies

Aqua Wiesbaden

Extremities

- CALLOSITIES, horny; Hands (17): **Am-c.**, ant-c., aq-gast., aq-wies., bor., calc-f., cist., **GRAPH.**, kali-ar., merc-i-r., nat-m., **Phos.**, posit., rhus-v., sil., **SULPH.**, thuj.

Carbons

Remedies: Graphites, Carbo vegetabilis, Glonoinum, Carboneum sulphuratum, Petroleum, Kreosotum.

Share and Compare Clinical Rubrics

Skin

- CICATRICES; cracked (4): aq-gast., crot-h., **Graph.**, *kali-c.*

Vertigo

- DEBAUCHERY, after (4): aq-gast., **Carb-v.**, coriand., nux-v.
- APOPLEXY, as before (6): aq-gast., **Glon.**, **Lach.**, ran-g., *sang.*, **Zinc.**

Male

- RETRACTION; scrotum (8): *acon.*, aloe, aq-gast., carbn-s., clem., lyss., petr., plb.

Face

- TUMOURS; lips (10): aq-gast., ars-i., **Con.**, cupre-l., galph., kreos., lap-a., phos., sep., vinc.

LAPIS ALBUS

Source

Calcium silicon-fluoride is a species of gneiss found in the mineral springs of Gastein where the waters flow over gneiss formations into a valley where goitre and cretinism abound.

Rubrics

Sensitivity and vulnerability: emotional and cognitive – loss of resilience – overwhelm

- SOMNAMBULISM; fasting, after (1): lap-a.

Clinical Rubric Clusters

Goitre and Thyroid dysfunction

Neck

- GOITRE; movable (1): **Lap-a.**
- GOITRE; soft (2): **Iod.**, lap-a.

- GOITER; painful (21) : am-c., bar-c., **Bell.**, brom., bry., caust., gamb., graph., **IOD.**, kali-i., lach., lap-a., **Merc.**, **Nat-ar.**, **Nat-c.**, nat-p., phos., **Plat.**, spong., sulph., **Zinc-i.**

Swelling Lymph Nodes – elastic

Clinical

- SWELLING; soft, elastic, lymphatic tissue, cervical (2): ail., *lap-a.*

Generalities

- SWELLING; soft; glands (2): kali-m., lap-a.
- SWELLING: elastic, would not pit (5): am-c., **ARS.**, conch., dor., lap-a.
- TUMOURS; lymphatic tissue, lymphangioma (15): am-m., ars-i., bar-c., bry., con., ho., iod., lap-a., phos., phyt., **Rad-br.**, **Sec.**, sil., sulph., **Vip.**

Neck

- STIFFNESS; cervical region; lymphatic tissue (3): astac., lach., lap-a.
- SWELLING; cervical region; lymphatic tissue; suppuration, in (2): cist., lap-a.

Cancer and Tumours (as supportive treatment)

Chest

- CANCER; soft and tender, mammae (4): calc-i., kali-chl., kali-m., lap-a.
- CANCER; ulcerating, mammae; painful (5): cadm., hippoz., lap-a., phyt., **Sil.**
- PAIN; constant; mammae (2): hep., **Lap-a.**

Female

- CANCER; painful, uterus (5): ars., bufo-s., **Carb-an.**, lap-a., **Sec.**
- HAEMORRHAGE, uterine, metrorrhagia; cancer of uterus, in (10): **Carb-an.**, **Kreos.**, **Lach.**, **Lap-a.**, **Med.**, **Nit-ac.**, **Phos.**, **Sec.**, THLASPI, Ust.

Face

- CANCER; cheeks (3): *ars.*, lap-a., syc-co.
- CANCER; jaw; lower (4): **Dulc.**, hecla., lap-a., thuj.
- TUMORS; jaw, lower, injury, after (1): lap-a.
- TUMOURS; red, hard, lower jaw (1): lap-a.
- TUMOURS; jaw, lower (5): amyg-p., astra-e., *hecla.*, lap-a., **Thuj.**
- TUMOURS; lips; lower (3): aq-gast., lap-a., phos.
- TUMOURS; lips (10): aq-gast., ars-i., **Con.**, cupre-l., galph., kreos., lap-a., phos., sep., vinc.

Generalities

- TUMOURS; fibroid; haemorrhage, with (11): calc., epih., **Hydrin-m.**, lap-a., nit-ac., phos., sabin., sul-ac., thlaspi, **Tril.**, ust.

Clinical

- TERMINAL diseases (22) : acet-ac., ars., ars-i., aster., bar-i., bar-m., cadm., calc-i., carb-ac., carb-an., carb-v., con., euph., hydr., kali-i., kreos., lap-a., merc., ph-ac., stann., tarent., tarent-c.

Tuberculosis (as supportive treatment)

Back

- SWELLING; tubercular, lymphatic tissue (3): ars-i., cist., lap-a.

Skin

- ABSCESSES, suppurations; tubercular (2): cist., lap-a.

Menses – Painful

Abdomen

- PAIN; menses; ameliorates (11): **Aster.**, bell., eupi., kali-c., kali-p., lac-c., **Lach.**, **Lap-a.**, mosch., sep., sulph.

Female

- MENSES; painful, dysmenorrhoea; fainting, with (15): aml-n., calc-f., **Cocc.**, **Cycl.**, **Kali-s.**, **Lach.**, **Lap-a.**, **Lyc.**, **Nux-m.**, **Nux-v.**, puls., **Sars.**, **Sep.**, tub., xan.
- PAIN; uterus; menses; beginning of (16): bor., **Calc.**, **Calc-p.**, caul., **Caust.**, graph., harp., **Kali-c.**, **Lach.**, **LAP-A.**, lyc., pitu-a., sile-c., tub., **Vib.**, wye.

Useful and/or Unusual Rubrics

Head

- PAIN, headache; fibrosis of uterus, with (2): **Lap-a.**, til.

Eyes

- INFLAMMATION; painless, iris (2): lap-a., merc-pr-r.
- INFLAMMATION; iris, iritis; left (4): **Cocc.**, **Hep.**, lap-a., *spig.*

Face

- WHITE; patches; cheeks, inner (2): **Am-caust.**, lap-a.
- WHITE; patches; cheeks, inner; left (1): lap-a.

Stomach

- PAIN; burning; pylorus (1): lap-a.
- PAIN; stitching; pylorus (1): lap-a.
- PAIN; stitching; cardiac orifice (3): *lact.*, lap-a., *sumb.*

Female

- PAIN; burning, smarting; fibrosis of uterus, with (1): **Lap-a**
- MENSES; irregular; girls, in young (3): lap-a., mill., senec.
- ITCHING; violent (21): *ambr.*, canth., caust., **CON.**, **Croto-t.**, goss., grat., hydrc., kreos., lac-f., **Lap-a.**, olea, **Petr.**, **Rhus-t.**, **Sec.**, sep., **Sol-t-ae.**, **SULPH.**, *tarent.*, tus-fa., xero.

Generalities

- FIBROSIS (5): calc-f., ion-rad., **Lap-a.**, thiosin., til.

AQUA TEPLITZ

Source

Water of the hot and alkaline mineral spring rising at Teplitz in Bohemia, Germany – flowing at 39 degrees Celsius.

Content

The remedy made from the water – contains:

- Row 2: Lithium carbonate, lithium chloride.
- Row 3: Sodium carbonate, sodium chloride, sodium fluoride, sodium silicate, aluminium oxide, silica.
- Row 4: Potassium chloride, potassium sulphate, calcium carbonate, calcium iodate, ferrous carbonate, ferrous fluorosilicate, manganese carbonate.
- Row 5: Strontium carbonate, strontium chloride.

Rubrics

Sensitivity and vulnerability: emotional and cognitive – loss of resilience – overwhelm

- DELUSIONS, imaginations; gave way; ground under him (4): aq-tep., cypra-e., digin., kali-br.
- DELUSIONS, imaginations; gave way; everything under him (5): aq-sanic., aq-tep., cypra-e., digin., kali-br.
- DELUSIONS, imaginations; legs; long, too (17): alum., aq-tep., aster., blatta, cann-i., carb-an., **Cinnb.**, **Coloc.**, haliae-lc., herin., **Kreos.**, lac-c., phos., **Rhus-t.**, stram., tab., thuj.

Clinical Rubric Clusters

Eruptions and Blue Penis and Blue Scrotum

Male

- BLUE; penis; glans (2): aq-tep., ars.
- BLUE; penis (5): aq-tep., **Arn.**, ars., merc-cy., sulph.
- BLUE; scrotum; eruptions, after (1): aq-tep.
- BLUE; scrotum (8): amyg-am., aq-tep., **ARN.**, **Ars.**, con., merc-cy., **Mur-ac.**, **Puls.**

- ABSCESSES, suppurations; penis; glans (3): aq-tep., merc., **Thuj.**
- PAIN; drawing; testes; right (12): acon., anag., aq-tep., **AUR.**, bry., mit., ol-an., raph., **RHOD.**, staph., tax., tus-p.

Eruptions

- Vesicular and painful – face and penis and scrotum – scrotum goes blue after eruptions.
- Pustules and erysipelas and military eruptions.

'Never Well Since' Vasectomy – drawing up, pain and recurrent swelling testes

Compare: Rhododendron

Male

- PAIN; drawing; spermatic cords; right (13): all-c., ammc., anag., aq-tep., arg., **Berb.**, *cassi-s.*, cimic., lact., nat-p., **Rhod.**, sabin., sulph.
- PAIN; drawing; testes; right (12): acon., anag., aq-tep., **AUR.**, bry., mit., ol-an., raph., **RHOD.**, staph., tax., tus-p.

- SWELLING; painful; testes (15): apis, aq-tep., **Arg.**, **Aur.**, benz., berb., **BROM.**, **Clem.**, colocin., **Dulc.**, **HAM.**, **Puls.**, Rhod., **SPONG.**, Thuj.

Rheumatic disorders

Joint Pain and Swelling and inflammation

Extremities; PAIN:

- Stitching; shoulders; alternating with shooting in elbows (1): aq-tep.
- Stitching; elbows; alternating with shooting in shoulders (1): aq-tep.
- Tearing; elbows; alternating with tearing in shoulders (1): aq-tep.
- Elbows; alternating with pain in; shoulders (2): aq-tep., kalm.
- Broken, as if; hips; walking, on (2): aq-tep., dros.
- Boring, digging; upper arms; bones, humerus (8): aq-tep., **Carb-v.**, cocc., kali-bi., **Mang.**, mang-acet., mel-alt., nat-c.
- Aching; thighs; bones, femur (9): aq-tep., bry., fl-ac., **IP.**, menis., **Merc-i-r.**, phos., plut-n., salx-p.
- Burning, smarting; elbows; bend of (9): aq-tep., kali-n., laur., led., nic-r., rat., rhus-v., sulph., teucr.
- Cutting; ankles; walking, while (5): aq-tep., benz-ac., cycl., iodof., polyp-p.
- Stitching; twitching; toes (7): aq-tep., berb., carbn-s., **Cina**, hell., kali-n., merl.
- Violent; shoulders; right (3): aq-tep., carb-ac., *chel.*
- Violent; wrists (5): act-sp., apoc-a., aq-tep., **Caul.**, hipp.
- STIFFNESS; shoulders; left (7): aids, aq-tep., bamb-a., guai., pull-g., salx-f., sep.

Back Pain

Aching, drawing, stitching and shooting – extending down back and down limbs, aggravated by motion and associated with constipation.

Back

- PAIN; cervical region; extending; back, down; lumbar region, to (4): aq-tep., ros-ca-a., stry., *verat.*
- PAIN; lumbar region, lumbago; constipation, with (4): **ALOE**, aq-tep., euon., kali-bi.
- PAIN; aching; lumbar region; constipation, with (2): aq-tep., kali-bi.

PAIN; lumbar region, lumbago; extending to:

- Abdomen; pelvis (6): aloe, androc., aq-tep., **BERB.**, eupi., laur.
- Calves (6): aq-tep., berb., ozone, ph-ac., pitu-a., zinc.

PAIN; corrosive, gnawing; dorsal region:

- Scapulae; between (2): aq-tep., *nat-c.*
- Scapulae (6): agar., alum., aq-tep., berb., nat-c., ph-ac.

- PAIN; drawing; lumbar region; extending to; calves (1): aq-tep. and pelvis (1): aq-tep.
- PAIN; tearing; drawing; scapulae (2): aq-tep., stann.

Paralysis – sensation of and actual

Generalities

- PARALYSIS; lower part, paraplegia; vertigo, with (3): aq-tep., bell., thuj.

Vertigo

- PARALYSIS; during (11): aq-tep., arg-n., **Arn.**, bapt., bell., **Caust.**, **Con.**, **GRAPH.**, **Nux-v.**, tep., thuj., **Zinc.**

Irritable bowel syndrome

Stomach

- PAIN; burning; drinks; ameliorate; cold (6): agar-em., apis, aq-tep., mangi., phos., pyrus-c.
- NAUSEA; constipation, with (16): aq-tep., asc-t., atista, buni-o., carb-v., *cinch.*, **COCC.**, cupr., dys-co., *gran.*, **Hyper.**, kurch., **Lac-d.**, *mag-c.*, still., tax-br.

Abdomen

- PAIN; inguinal region; extending to; back; spine (1): aq-tep.
- PAIN; stitching; inguinal region; extending to; spine (1): aq-tep.
- PAIN; stitching; hypochondria; inspiration, on; deep (8): aq-tep., aur., **Bell.**, **Calc-p.**, form., nat-s., ol-an., sil.
- PAIN; inguinal region; extending to; back (12): am-m., aq-tep., arg., bor., carb-v., cast., daph., mag-m., mobil-ph., nit-ac., sep., **Sulph.**
- PAIN; tearing; menses; before (3): aq-tep., **Cinnb.**, nat-m.
- PAIN; hypogastrium; haemorrhage, with uterine (6): acet-ac., aq-tep., chin., hydr., mag-c., **Sec.**

Rectum

- ERUPTIONS; itching; perineum (3): alum., aq-tep., morg.
- ERUPTIONS; perineum (9): aq-tep., brom., graph., med., **Morg.**, **Petr.**, sars., **Sulph.**, tell.
- MUCOUS: white (2): aq-tep., plect. and acrid, excoriating (4): aq-tep., chin., phos., **Thuj.**

- MOISTURE; acrid, corrosive, excoriating (12): aq-tep., ars-s-f., **Carb-v.**, chin., lach., **Merc-c.**, **Nit-ac.**, **Nux-v.**, **Paeon.**, phos., **Thuj.**, *zinc.*

Useful and or Unusual Rubrics

Generalities

- PAIN; piercing; iron, as from a hot (4): aq-tep., **Alum.**, *cann-i.*, vesp.
- HAEMORRHAGE; ameliorates; haemorrhoids, of (1): aq-tep.

Extremities; COLDNESS, chilliness:

- Hips; deep seated (1): aq-tep.
- Thighs; bones, femur (1): aq-tep.
- Painful; thighs, femur (1): aq-tep.
- Painful; lower limbs (4): aq-tep., caust., chel., **Syph.**
- Internal (6): aq-tep., cass., helo., quas., **Rhus-t.**, *ruta.*
- Wind, as from; upper arms (2): aq-tep., nat-m.
- Wind, as from; upper limbs (6): aq-tep., aster., m-aust., mosch., nat-m., *rhus-t.*

Vertigo

- OBJECTS seem; move, to; houses, while walking (1): aq-tep.

Head

- CONGESTION, hyperaemia; weakness, with (3): apis, aq-tep., **Tab.**

PAIN, headache:

- Drawing; forehead; extending to; jaw, lower (3): aq-tep., nat-m., rhus-t.
- Forehead; extending; face, to; jaw, to; lower (6): aq-tep., bell., brom., cath-a., nat-m., rhus-t.
- Sore, bruised; scalp, external; touching hair aggravates (6): **Alum.**, aq-tep., lycpr., salx-n., **Sil.**, **Spig.**

Eyes

- PAIN; cramping; lids; upper (3): agar., aq-tep., **Stram.**
- ERYSIPELAS; lids (6): **Apis**, aq-tep., calc-i., **Hep.**, rhus-t., tep., vesp.

Ears

- OBSTRUCTION, obstructed sensation; perspiration, as from (1): aq-tep.
- PAIN; tearing; coals, as from glowing (1): aq-tep.
- SWELLING; concha (7): ant-c., aq-tep., arn., nat-m., phos., sil., spong.

Face

- ERUPTIONS; rash; miliary, chin (1): aq-tep.

- ERUPTIONS; rash; chin (8): aids, am-c., aq-mar., aq-tep., coriand., **Dulc.**, nic-r., syph.
- WHITE; chin, spots, after scratching (1): aq-tep.

- DISTORTION; one-sided (6): aq-tep., *hyos.*, *merc.*, *nux-v.*, **Syph.**, tell.

Mouth

- ERUPTIONS; vesicles; tongue; root, base (4: aq-tep., canth., cocc., *graph.*
- HAEMORRHAGE; frequent, gums (4): aq-tep., *bar-c.*, **Carb-v.**, lach.
- PROTRUDING; convulsive, spasmodic, tongue (4): aq-tep., cina, cocc., sec.

Teeth

- PAIN, toothache; piercing; iron, as with a hot (1): aq-tep.
- PAIN, toothache; boring; molars, bicuspids; upper (3): aq-tep., kali-c., seneg.

Throat

- PAIN; inflammation, without (1): aq-tep.

Neck

- PAIN; stitching; extending to; ear (5): alum., aq-tep., hep., hydrog., phos.

Female

- LEUCORRHEA; Starch, like boiled (6): aq-tep., **BOR.**, cur., ferr-i., lach., **NAT-M.**, **SABIN.**

Larynx and trachea

- PAIN; larynx; swallowing; ameliorates (3): aq-tep., spig., tarax.

Speech and voice

- DIFFICULT speech; convulsions, spasms of organs, from; tongue, of (8): **Agar.**, aq-tep., arg-n., cypr., lyc., **Ruta**, sec., **Stram.**

Respiration

- PAIN; from; abdomen, in; inguinal region (1): aq-tep.
- PAIN; from; throat, in (2): aq-tep., olnd.

Expectoration

- ERUPTIONS ameliorate (1): aq-tep.

Chest

- PAIN; stitching; needles, as from; mammae; right (2): adam., aq-tep.
- PAIN; stitching; needles, as from; mammae (9): adam., aq-tep., carb-an., con., grat., iod., kali-bi., ol-an., plb.

PAIN; tearing; muscles:

- Pectoral; extending to; shoulder (1): aq-tep.
- Pectoral (6): aq-tep., berb., merc., ran-a., *spig.*, til.

- TUMOURS; mammae; right (9): aq-tep., aster., bell., carc., con., lap-be-e., phel., *phyt.*, psor.
- TUMOURS; painful, mammae (9): aq-tep., berb-a., **Brom.**, calc-i., **Chim.**, **Con.**, phase., **Phyt.**, **Sil.**

Heart and circulation

- PAIN; stitching; heart region; palpitations, with (7): aq-tep., coff., hep., ign., lycps., myric., neod-n.
- PAIN; stitching; synchronous with pulse, heart region (8): aq-tep., both-a., dig., digin., iber., **Rhus-t.**, **SPIG.**, zinc.

Extremities

- ABSCESSES, suppurations; elbows (4): aq-tep., crot-h., dros., sil.
- ABSCESSES, suppurations; legs (8): anth., aq-tep., both-l., calc., chin., guai., psor., sulph.
- ERUPTIONS; rash; shoulders (6): *amet.*, aq-tep., berb., **Calc.**, naja-m., puls.

- MOTION, motions; impossible; wrists (1): aq-tep.
- PARALYSIS; shoulders (12): aq-tep., **Arn.**, bell., **Caust.**, **Cur.**, **Ferr.**, ign., *lach.*, plb., puls., **RHUS-T.**, verat.

- CRAMPS; thighs; sleep; falling asleep, on (1): aq-tep.
- CRAMPS; legs; calves; sleep; during (12): adam., ant-t., aq-tep., coca, diox., echis-c., graph., inul., **Kali-c.**, *lach.*, nat-m., *sulph.*
- JERKING; toes; first (4): agar., aq-tep., ph-ac., puls.
- JERKING; legs; calves (10): act-sp., anac., aq-tep., cupr., cymbo-ci., **Graph.**, **Jatr.**, mag-m., **OP.**, *tarax.*

- HEAVINESS, weariness; lower limbs; constipation, with (1): aq-tep.

PAIN; tearing; muscles:

- Pectoral; extending to; shoulder (1): aq-tep.
- Pectoral (6): aq-tep., berb., merc., ran-a., *spig.*, til.

Related and Compare Remedies

Aqua

Remedies: Aqua Sanicula, Aqua Marina, Aqua Lippspringe, Aqua Wiesbaden.

- DELUSIONS, imaginations; gave way; everything under him (5): aq-sanic., aq-tep., cypra-e., digin., kali-br.

Face

- ERUPTIONS; rash; chin (8): aids, am-c., aq-mar., aq-tep., coriand., **Dulc.**, nic-r., syph.

Larynx and trachea

- MUCOUS in air passages; tenacious; trachea (7): aq-lipp., aq-tep., **Bry.**, **Cann-s.**, just., **Nux-v.**, vinc.

Generalities

- HAEMORRHAGE; ameliorates; anus, from (5): aesc., aq-tep., aq-wies., calad., ovi-g-p.

AQUA VICHY GRANDE GRILLE

Source

The Grande-grille mineral spring at Vichy in France – the largest of the hot springs arising in the spa town of Vichy at 39 degrees Celsius. There are several springs at Vichy, hot, warm and cold. Vichy water, a naturally sparkling cold spring bottled water continues to be popular in France.

Contents

- Row 2: Carbonic acid.
- Row 3: Sodium and magnesium salts – carbonate, chloride, phosphate and sulphate; hydrochloric acid, sulphuric acid, silica, phosphoric acid.
- Row 4: Potassium and calcium salts as carbonate, chloride, phosphate and sulphate; ferrous oxide and arsenic acid.

Proving

No proving details available. Symptoms gathered from patients bathing in the spa pool and drinking the water.

Sensitivity and vulnerability: emotional and cognitive – loss of resilience – overwhelm

- ANXIETY; future, about; morning (3): aq-vichy-g., mant-r., nabal.
- RESTLESSNESS, nervousness; dinner; ameliorates (2): aq-vichy-g., thuj.
- SADNESS; misfortune, as from (26): alum., apei-s., **Aq-Sanic.**, aq-vichy-g., aster., bros-g., **Calc.**, calc-acet., calc-s., **Chin-s.**, cycl., dros., hura, lyss., mez., **Naja**, ph-ac., phel., phos., plac., puls., rhus-t., sol, staph., sulph., **VERAT.**

Rubrics

Suppression of Emotion – Sublimation of libido

Abdomen

- RESTLESSNESS; waking, on (1): aq-vichy-g.

Rectum

- RESTLESSNESS: flatus aggravates (2): aq-vichy-g., chion.

Taste

- BITTER; morning; rising; aggravates (1): aq-vichy-g.

Water and Thirst and Dryness

Taste

- BITTER; thirst; with (4): aq-vichy-g., arist-m., gink., pic-ac.

Clinical Rubric Clusters

Body Odour

Smell

- CORPSE, like a; morning, on rising (1): aq-vichy-g.
- CORPSE, like a (3): aq-vichy-g., **Bell.**, chin.

Cucumbers – olfactory as if/illusion/delusion

Smell

- CUCUMBERS (1): aq-vichy-g.
- CUCUMBERS; morning (1): aq-vichy-g.

Irritable bowel syndrome

Stomach

- PAIN; burning; salivation, with (3): aq-vichy-g., *brom.*, *ter.*
- PAIN; salivation, with (12): aq-vichy-g., arn., bar-c., brom., *calc.*, caust., *croto-t.*, *gamb.*, *nat-c.*, *plat.*, *tab.*, ter.
- PAIN; burning; afternoon (16: alum., am-m., aq-vichy-g., bamb-a., *bar-c.*, bell., card-*b.*, fago., iris, kali-bi., lyc., lycpr., ol-an., olea, pyrus-c., *valer.*

Abdomen

PAIN

- Chocolate; ameliorates, flavoured with cinnamon (1): aq-vichy-g.
- Cramping, gripping; chocolate flavoured with cinnamon ameliorates (1): aq-vichy-g.

- DISTENSION; waking, on (3): aq-vichy-g., galph., ptel.
- PAIN; Morning; stool; ameliorates (6): aq-vichy-g., ars., ferr., indg., mez., phys.

PAIN; cramping, gripping:

- Alternating with; stitching below mastoid (1): aq-vichy-g.
- Morning; rising; on (8): aq-vichy-g., digin., ham., nat-m., ruta, trif-p., *trom.*, **Zinc-val.**

PAIN; diarrhoea would appear, as if:

- Afternoon; four p.m. (1): aq-vichy-g.
- Afternoon (3): aq-vichy-g., nat-c., nat-s.
- Evening (7): aq-vichy-g., cund., digin., iris-foe., mag-s., ph-ac., piloc.

Abdomen

- PAIN; pressing; hypochondria; extending; inward (2): aq-vichy-g., *sul-ac.*
- PAIN; pressing; (3): aq-vichy-g., ph-ac., spig.
- PAIN; stitching; gripping; morning, stool ameliorates (1): aq-vichy-g.
- PAIN; stitching; gripping (7): aq-vichy-g., bry., cann-s., carb-v., chin., spig., viol-t.

RUMBLING noise

- Daytime (5): agath-a., aq-vichy-g., cench., nit-ac., ptel.
- Burning (2): aq-vichy-g., asc-t.
- Colic; during (5): aq-vichy-g., **Dulc.**, **PULS.**, rham-cath., til.

Rectum

- FLATUS; burning (8): alf., **ALOE**, aq-vichy-g., asc-t., **Mag-m.**, **Plb-acet.**, psor., toxop-p.

Useful and/or Unusual Rubrics

Head

- ITCHING; morning; aggravates; rising, on (1): aq-vichy-g.

PAIN, headache

- Pressing; occiput; fever, during (3): aq-vichy-g., rhus-t., term-a.
- Stitching; occiput; protuberance (3): aq-vichy-g., nit-ac., pimp.
- Stitching; occiput; protuberance; left (1): aq-vichy-g.

Eyes

- PAIN; Stitching; lachrymation, with (7): aq-vchy-g., cyg-c., mag-m., mag-s., nat-c., petr., puls.

Vision

- SPARKS; variegated (2): aq-vichy-g., *stry*.
- VARIEGATED colours; sparks (2): aq-vichy-g., *galv*.
- SPARKS; morning (4): aq-vichy-g., calc., ferr-i., harp.

Ears

- PAIN; stitching; below (16): apis, aq-vichy-g., arist-cl., *bar-acet.*, bar-c., bry., coc-c., *croto-t.*, erio., hell., *mag-s.*, nit-ac., olnd., *sars.*, *viol-o.*, xan.

Nose

- CORYZA; cough; after (5): aq-vichy-g., bad., **Bell.**, **Hep.**, *kali-n.*

Face

- ERUPTIONS; pimples; painful; lip, upper (2): aq-vichy-g., **Sil.**
- ERUPTIONS; pimples; red; lip, upper (3): aq-vichy-g., posit., zinc.

- PAIN; pressing; eyes; below; left, after breakfast (1): aq-vichy-g.
- PAIN; stitching; jaws; articulation and left temple, between (1): aq-vichy-g.
- PAIN; twisting; jaw, lower (1): aq-vichy-g.
- PAIN; twisting (2): aq-vichy-g., paraf.
- SWELLING; sensation of; jaws; lower (2): aq-vichy-g., *sabad.*

Abdomen

- ENLARGED; liver; malaria, in or after (4): aq-vichy-g., *chion.*, *cory.*, merc-i-r.

Bladder

- PAIN; gripping; morning (1): aq-vichy-g.
- PAIN; gripping (5): aq-vichy-g., calc., **Coloc.**, mez., valer.

Urethra

- ITCHING; fossa navicularis (12): agar., aq-vichy-g., cic., **Clem.**, cocc., **Colch.**, *cub.*, ferr., gins., **PETROS.**, sulph., **Thuj.**

Male

- ITCHING; penis; glans; tip (14): *ang.*, *ant-c.*, aq-vichy-g., ars., blatta-a., calc., **Cinnb.**, coloc., ferr-m., *ferr-ma.*, nat-m., *sel.*, spong., thuj.

Respiration

- OPPRESSION, from; chest, in; load on, as from a (7): aq-vichy-g., *cina*, **Nux-m.**, rheum, sabad., spig., viol-o.

Cough

- DRY; tickling, from; throat, in (10): *am-m.*, aq-lipp., aq-vichy-g., crot-c., **Kali-c.**, **Phos.**, plut-n., sang., sid-al., zinc-i.

Chest

- BAR sensation, iron; extending across centre of chest (8): *aq-vichy-g.*, ars., **Haem.**, kali-bi., ox-ac., ran-s., ser-ang., *tab.*

PAIN; stitching; sternum; costal cartilages:

- False ribs, with; right (1): aq-vichy-g.
- False ribs, with (7): aq-vichy-g., carbn-s., cina, olnd., plat., staph., sul-ac.

- PAIN; tearing; sternum; costal cartilages with false ribs (3): aq-vichy-g., grat., merc-c.
- PAIN; stitching; Heart region; sitting, while (8): aq-vichy-g., calc-f., fago., gink., *mur-ac.*, *rhus-t.*, valer., viol-t.

Back

- PAIN; stitching; lumbar region; right (13): *ammc.*, aq-vichy-g., bor., bos-s., caj., **Coloc.**, hydrc., lyc., oryc-c., pimp., **Ran-b.**, sep., til.
- STIFFNESS; cervical region; muscles; scaleni, left, afternoon, after false step (1): aq-vichy-g.
- STIFFNESS; painful; motion aggravates (8): aq-vichy-g., cinch., *cocc.*, dros., **Guai.**, **Led.**, **Mez.**, rhus-t.
- STIFFNESS; cervical region; muscles (11): ap-g., aq-calc-caust., aq-vichy-g., bung-f., **Cham.**, *cocc.*, hura, imp-w., iris, lac-f., meteo-a.

Extremities

- PAIN; feet; extending to; tibia (3): aq-vichy-g., bamb-a., nat-m.
- PAIN; stitching; feet; back; extending to tibia (1): aq-vichy-g.
- PAIN; stitching; feet; back; right (6): aq-vichy-g., canth., colocin., ferr., galph., iodof.

Generalities

- FOOD and drinks; chocolate; ameliorates (5): aq-vichy-g., arge-p., calc-s., cordy-a., helod-c.
- PAIN; gripping, grasping, clawing; morning (4): aq-vichy-g., petr., *puls.*, sulph.

Compare and Related Remedies

Aqua

Remedies: Aqua Sanicula, Aqua Lippspringe.

Rectum

- URGING, desire; flatus; aggravates (9): **ALOE**, **Aq-Sanic.**, aq-vichy-g., hedeo., nat-s., **Nux-v.**, oxyg., ruta, spig.

Cough

- DRY; tickling, from; throat, in (10): *am-m.*, aq-lipp., aq-vichy-g., crot-c., **Kali-c.**, **Phos.**, plut-n., sang., sid-al., zinc-i.

Acids – compare at Clinical Rubric Level

Remedies: Nitric acid, Picric acid, Sulphuric acid, Phosphoric acid and Gallic acids.

Head

- PAIN, headache; Stitching; occiput; protuberance (3): aq-vichy-g., nit-ac., pimp.

Taste

- BITTER; thirst; with (4): aq-vichy-g., arist-m., gink., pic-ac.

Abdomen

- PAIN; pressing; hypochondria; extending; inward (2): aq-vichy-g., *sul-ac.*
- PAIN; cramping, gripping (3): aq-vichy-g., ph-ac., spig.

Rectum

- RESTLESSNESS (13): aq-vich-g., chion., dios., gall-ac., haliae-lc., **Iris**, kali-c., lyc., med., nux-v., plan., sin-n., sumb.

Spigelia anthelmia – compare at clinical rubric level

Face

- PAIN; jaws; lower; chewing; aggravates (6): aegle-f., aq-vichy-g., ph-ac., posit., *spig.*, verat.
- PAIN; pressing; eyes; below (7): act-sp., aq-vichy-g., *ars.*, *cina*, lac-v-b., *spig.*, *spong.*

Abdomen

- PAIN; cramping, gripping; pressive (3): aq-vichy-g., ph-ac., spig.
- PAIN; stitching; gripping (7): aq-vichy-g., bry., cann-s., carb-v., chin., spig., viol-t.

References

1 La Moreaux PE, Turner, J. *Springs and bottled waters of the world: Ancient history, source, occurrence, quality and use.* Berlin: Springer-Verlag, 2001.
2 O'Hare JP. *et al.* Physiology of Immersion in Thermal waters. In: Kellaway GA (ed). *Hot Springs of Bath Investigations of the Thermal Waters of the Avon Valley.* Bath: Bath City Council, 1991. pp. 71–76.
3 Edmunds WM, Miles DL. The geochemistry of Bath Thermal Waters. In: Kellaway GA (ed). *Hot Springs of Bath Investigations of the Thermal Waters of the Avon Valley.* Bath: Bath City Council, 1991. pp. 143–156.
4 Sevar R. The water of the Cross Spring in Bath – a homeopathic proving. *Homeopathic Links*, 2002; 15(03): 183–188.
5 Andrews, J.N. Radioactivity and Dissolved Gases. In: Kellaway GA (ed). *Hot Springs of Bath Investigations of the Thermal Waters of the Avon Valley.* Bath: Bath City Council, 1991. pp. 157–170.

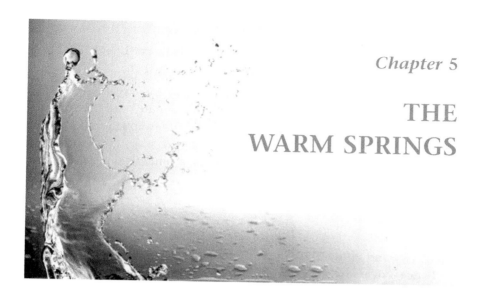

THE
WARM SPRINGS

The Warm Springs included in this book are: Aqua Narzan, Aqua Reinerz and Aqua Sanicula.

AQUA NARZAN

Source

Rising at the foot of the Caucasus Mountains near the town of Kiszlavodsk in Russia, one of the springs remains the most popular bottled sparkling water in Russia. Half a million people visit the area every year for treatment, rest and recreation.

History

The water of the 14 springs of Narzan have been recognised as having medicinal properties and been drunk and bathed in since 1717. Kiszlavodsk has the highest recorded number of sunny days of any town in Russia.

Content

Aqua Narzan spring contains 2.3 grams of minerals per litre, pH 6.2 and flows at 14 degrees Celsius, even in the Russian winter.

- Row 2: Carbon dioxide, carbonic acid, nitrogen and oxygen.
- Row 3: Sodium sulphate, magnesium carbonate and magnesium bicarbonate, magnesium chloride, magnesium sulphate, aluminium phosphate, silica.
- Row 4: Potassium sulphate, calcium carbonate, and calcium bicarbonate, ferrous carbonate, manganese carbonate.

Rubrics

Sensitivity and vulnerability: emotional and cognitive – loss of resilience – overwhelm

- Excitable and ailments from over-excitement.
- Sensation as if intoxicated – pleasant.
- Sensation as if warmth all over the body – feet warm in the afternoon.
- Inclination to perspire.
- Desire to smoke tobacco or sudden aversion.
- Aversion to previously desired foods.
- Pains: biting, corroding, darting, lightning, quick, shooting, stitching.

Tension – mind and body

- Contraction of penis and contraction of skin glans penis – cannot retract the foreskin.
- Pain in spermatic cord.
- Hiccoughs and Heartburn and Eructation and Flatulence after bread or acid drinks.
- Urging to stool but only flatulence is passed with stitching pains in abdomen.
- Pain in back as if sprained, worse moving about and worse coughing.

Water and Thirst

- Thirsty for water.
- Constant sensation of dryness in throat and desire to drink water.
- Restless sleep because of insistent thirst and dryness in throat.
- Thirst and dryness of throat waking him throughout the night – obliged to rise and drink water.

Exhaustion – mental and physical

- Sensation as if feet are weary as after a long walk.
- Sensitivity of the heels and bruised pain in feet.
- Indifference and apathy.
- Weariness and weakness and sleepiness.

Suppression of Emotion – Sublimation of libido

Male

- CONTRACTION; penis (6): aq-narz., asar., chin., ign., plb., puls.

Compare/Related Remedies

Croton tiglium

Male

- PAIN; corrosive, gnawing (8): agn., aq-narz., calad., **CROTO-T.**, nux-v., ph-ac., plat., plb.
- PAIN; corrosive, gnawing: Scrotum (3): aq-narz., **CROTO-T.**, plat.
- PAIN; corrosive, gnawing: Penis (6): agn., aq-narz., calad., croto-t., nux-v., plb.

Useful and/or Unusual Rubrics

Male; PAIN; biting:

- Scrotum (6): aq-narz., hep., *her-s.*, ol-an., plat., *ran-s.*
- Penis (21): aq-narz., *bell.*, bor., calad., chin-s., coc-c., cop., **Hep.**, ign., kali-c., m-arct., m-art., merc., nat-c., nat-m., *nux-v.*, *phos.*, plb., puls., thuj., *viol-t.*

Stool

- WATERY; hiccough, in (1): aq-narz.

AQUA REINERZ

Source

A warm spring at Reinerz in Wabrzych-Klodzko geothermal region of southern Poland.

Content

- Row 3: Sodium carbonate, sodium chloride, magnesium carbonate, silica, and phosphoric acid.
- Row 4: Potassium sulphate, calcium carbonate, ferrous carbonate, ferrous oxide, manganese carbonate and manganese arsenate.

Proving

Symptoms are from bathing in and drinking the water and from cured cases.

Rubrics

Clinical Rubric Cluster – irritable bowel syndrome

Abdomen

- DISTENSION; motion; ameliorates; constant (1): aq-rein.
- DISTENSION; motion; ameliorates (7): aq-rein., aran-ix., chin., kali-c., mand., *op.*, *phos.*
- FULLNESS; stool; ameliorates (2): aq-rein., colch.

- DISTENSION; stool; ameliorates (24): alum., am-m., aq-rein., asaf., calc-p., chir-f., cinis-p., corn., falco-p., haliae-lc., hema-h., hyper., lam-cy., lat-h., meteo-a., nat-c., nat-m., onc-t., paraf., phos., ros-ca-a., sulph., telo-s., **Thuj.**

AQUA SANICULA

Source

A warm and bubbly spring in Ottawa, Illinois.

History

The water was used in the 19th century as a spa, sold as naturally sparkling medicinal spring water and used to produce ginger ale and birch beer – the spring was permanently sealed beneath a concrete wall after the Starved Rock Dam was completed in 1933.

Contents

Constituents of the water:

- Row 2: Lithium bicarbonate, borax.
- Row 3: Sodium chloride, sodium bicarbonate, sodium bromide, sodium iodide, sodium phosphate, magnesium chloride, aluminium oxide, silica.
- Row 4: Calcium bicarbonate, calcium chloride, calcium sulphate, ferrous bicarbonate.

Provings[1]

- In potencies by Dr Martin Deshere in 1867 using trituration of the evaporated water.
- Dr JG. Grunlach and his family, who drank the water for a year and suffered from the symptoms, periodically, for the rest of their lives.

Rubrics

Sensitivity and vulnerability: emotional and cognitive – loss of resilience – overwhelm

- Sensation of impending doom and misfortune.
- Sensation as if everything is giving way beneath her and vertex would fly off – dread of downward motion – motion sickness.
- Dream of robbers – house must be searched.
- Constant irresistible desire to look behind her when walking.
- Sees people behind him when walking in the dark.
- Great fear of darkness.

- Sensation as if no one admires her and everyone hates her.
- Misconstrues actions and motives of others.
- Feels forsaken – yet wants nothing to do with anyone – doesn't want to be touched – can't bear to have one part of body touch another – must hold fingers apart – sweats where parts of body touch one another.

- Stubborn and Contrary and Capricious.
- Headstrong and obstinate.
- Contrary – refuses to do everything asked of them will only do the opposite or only exactly what they want.
- Irritable and angry – children cry and kick and throw self-backward (like Chamomilla).
- Capricious: ask for things then throw away, don't know what they want.

- Trifling symptoms are unbearable – yet at other times may not complain even when in pain or very ill.

Restlessness

- Child desires to be carried and carried quickly – yet may still arch backwards (like Chamomilla).
- No stability of purpose – constantly changing interests and occupation – mind wanders from subject to subject.
- Restless desire to go from place to place yet not ameliorated by motion or travel and when ill is much worse from jarring.
- Restless until exhausted.
- Motion sickness – nausea and vomiting from car or train or boat yet thirsty.

Fears

- Dark.
- Downward motion and falling – children cling to mother.
- Robbers.
- Someone behind them.
- Something bad will happen.
- Being medically examined – resists.

Modalities and Food

- Aggravation: downward motion, jarring, straining at stool, cold wind on occiput or neck.
- Ameliorated by: open air, warmth, uncovering, being carried quickly.
- Desires: bacon, ham, ham fat, milk, sweet, salt.
- Averse fish.

Related remedies – see after the clinical cases

Clinical

Odour of fish or fish brine or odour of strong or rotten cheese

- Orifices and mucous membranes and breath.
- Discharges and stools.
- Perforated eardrum which will not heal.

Constipation

- Huge stool difficult to pass and painful or causing anal fissure.
- Bashful stool – partially emerges and then recedes.
- Stool as if cut with a knife (lengthways) and square stool.

Exhaustion – mental and physical

Weight loss and failure to thrive and progressive emaciation – child becomes extremely thin and looks old and wrinkled – skin hangs in folds.

Useful rubrics in children

- Head; HARD; baby in, no sign suture or posterior fontanel.
- FONTANELS; closing premature, prior to birth.
- HEAT; tongue; stick it out, has to, to cool it.
- Stool; SQUARE; carved with a knife, as if.
- Expectoration; CHEESE; like, large, sinking in water.
- FOOD and DRINKS: bread; desires; fresh only.
- FOOD + DRINKS: milk; desires; icy cold.

Unique rubrics

Mind

- DELUSIONS, imaginations; Gave way; everything under him.
- IRRITABILITY; Alternating with; playfulness.
- KICKS; Nine pm. – midnight.
- SHRIEKING, screaming, shouting; Night; nine pm. – midnight.
- TOUCHED; Aversion of being; cannot bear anyone to lie close to or touch him.
- WEEPING, tearful mood; Children, in; laughing aggravates.

Vertigo

- KNEADING bread or making similar motions.
- RIDING on horseback; aggravates; in dark.
- SPINE; as if vertebrae gliding over each other; lumbar region, rocking in a chair.

Head

- ELECTRICAL hair; Crackling when combed.
- FLY off, as if vertex would; Motion, from downward.

Eyes

- ULCERS; Lids; margins, edges; lower.

Mouth

- HEAT; Tongue; stick it out, has to, to cool it.
- SALIVA; Viscid; cutting teeth, when.
- SALIVA; White; cutting teeth, when.
- ULCERS; Palate; centre; food and drinks, warm, aggravate.

Teeth

- PAIN; Pulled out, as if; left in their sockets, and.
- THIN, as if.

Throat

- CHOKING, constricting; Bread crumbs, as from.

Abdomen

- PAIN; Umbilicus; region of; eruptions around umbilicus, before.

Rectum

- INVOLUNTARY stool; Cross legs, must.
- URGING, desire; Flatus; for; cross legs, must, to prevents escaping.

Female

- OPEN; Uterus; os uteri; three weeks before delivery, parturition.
- PAIN; Bearing down; uterus and region of; rest ameliorates; jar, misstep aggravates; lying ameliorates; rest ameliorates.

Respiration

- ASTHMATIC; Supper, after.
- WHEEZING, whistling; Eating, during or after.
- RATTLING; Eating, during or after.

Expectoration

- CARTILAGE, like boiled.
- CHEESE, like; Large, sinking in water.

Back

- COLDNESS, chilliness; Spine; motion; ameliorates; sitting still, on; warmth ameliorates.
- GLIDING over each other, as if, vertebrae; Lumbar, rocking in a chair.
- PAIN; Broken, as if; lumbar region; morning; rising, on.
- PAIN; Burning; lumbar and sacral regions; exercise, gentle, ameliorates; and lying; flat on back ameliorates.
- STIFFNESS; Morning; strain, after.
- STIFFNESS: Turns whole body to look around.
- WEAKNESS; Walking; while; snow, over.

Extremities

- ERUPTIONS; Moist; toes.
- PAIN; Feet; soles; uncover, inclination to.
- PAIN; Rheumatic; shoulders; heat ameliorates, sits with back to fire.

- PERSPIRATION; Stepped in cold water, as if, feet, soles.
- SWELLING; Hands; pregnancy, in.

Chill

- PERIODICAL; Regular and distinct; every day.

Skin

- ERUPTIONS; Boils, furuncles; maturing; not.

Generals

- MOTION; aggravates; during; arms of; kneading bread or making similar motion.

CASE 5.1 A child with cancer

Context

G is a beautiful girl of almost 5 years old with lovely big green eyes. She is very tall and very thin, is bald and has no eyebrows or eyelashes.

Consultation 28th February 2005

She was well till 23rd November 2004 when her left leg became very swollen and she went into hospital for tests. They found a large tumour in her left pelvis. She had a biopsy which showed a desmoplastic small round cell tumour compressing her iliac vessels. There was a secondary in the right side of the pelvis but no spread to bones or liver or lungs. She has an in-dwelling central venous line and is having her stem cells harvested. She has been on very intensive chemotherapy since December in 3 weeks cycles – vincristine, doxyrubicin, phosphamide and something else I can't remember.

She was 20 kg and now she is 17.3 kg. She gets terrible side-effects from the chemotherapy – nausea and vomiting and a very sore mouth and her whole gastro-intestinal lining gets sore and ulcerated. She has no interest in food as her mouth is so sore from the ulcers and she gets a fear of eating and avoids it because of the pain on swallowing. She needs an operation in 3 weeks to de-bulk and hopefully remove the tumour which has been responding well to chemotherapy. She had 4 very traumatic attempts to place a central venous line and needed 4 general anaesthetics with gas so she has a fear of hospitals. We give her daily injections through her venous line of a bone marrow stimulant to aid her recovery. She has had a lot of blood transfusions and platelet transfusions and such a lot of intravenous antibiotics and anti-fungal drugs.

She is so very constipated. Before she got ill she usually had 2 bowels motions a day but now she can go a week without producing anything. And when it does come out it is hard lumps like round dark balls like rabbit droppings. And sometimes the stool is so huge and it hurts her and sometimes it seems to come half out and then slip back in again. The stools are very dense large lumps. Sometimes they look like they have been cut with a knife.

She is on ondancitron for the nausea and recently metoclopramide. The nausea is worse in the morning. She eats a bit more in the afternoon and evening. She gags easily and she wakens at night with a cough or wakens to pass urine and then she usually vomits.

On days 7 to 14 of the chemo cycles she gets lots of mouth ulcers and can't open her mouth or stick her tongue out. The ulcers are huge – about 2 cm and shallow with well defined edges. She has lots of saliva – it just pours out of her mouth because she can't swallow it with the pain. Yes, she is still growing well – she has grown 7 to 8 cm since she has been ill.

There is cancer on my side of the family (mother): her maternal grandmother and grandfather and my sister.

She is usually warm and strips her clothes off when she is too hot. She would wear a skirt and a swimsuit in the snow if I let her. When she is ill she gets burning hot hands. She doesn't sweat much even with a fever, but she will sweat if she gets angry or worried. She has never had a high fever since being ill – they give her antibiotics if her axilla temperature goes above 36 degrees.

She hates vegetables – hates anything green, and she doesn't like sweets or chocolate. She loves some things for a while and then goes off them: salmon, tomato soup, bran flakes, egg yolks, cooked ham, olives, beetroot, fruit juice and recently Coke. She is not thirsty.

She is very strong willed, extremely stubborn and so obstinate. She is very determined even to her own detriment – she will have things her way or not at all. Recently she has been more aggressive – if she doesn't get her own way she will lash out and hit me or her brother. She is my first child. Yes my first pregnancy. She is vain and loves to dress up as a fairy princess. If she is told off she hates it – she gets sad and reacts and hits and says "don't tell me off."

She has had bad reactions to some drugs. She got agitated with lorazepam. She was on 30 mg of morphine and she went into a cold turkey reaction when they abruptly stopped it. She has been in and out of hospital so much.

Analysis

This is the first child with cancer that I've treated with homeopathy. The role of homeopathy is supportive – all her conventional treatment must continue – this is already clear to me and her mother.

Since there is a clear picture of a remedy I recognize I agree to begin treatment.

How is her vitality? It must be good to have survived recurrent bacterial and fungal septicaemia.

Are there obstacles to healing? She has needed so many courses of intravenous antibiotics and anti-fungal drugs to save her life – she is clearly immune-suppressed from the chemotherapy and will have an abnormal bowel flora which adds to immune suppression – she needs a bowel nosode.

Since she cannot eat properly she needs nutritional supplements until she can.

Rubrics – retrospective

- Generalities; cancerous affections.
- Obstinate, headstrong; children (40).**
- Capriciousness.**
- Capriciousness; children, in (9).
- Irritability; children, in.*
- Kicks.*
- Rectum; constipation; stool; recedes (34).
- Rectum; constipation; stool; remains long in rectum with (40).
- Stool; large.

The repoeratorisation matrix generated by MacRepertory using Complete Repertory 2015 by Van Zandvoot[2] (Figure 5.1), shows Aqua Sanicula has all her clear mind symptoms and her functional bowel symptoms.

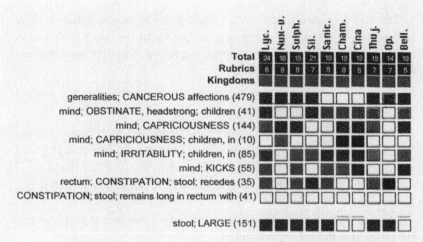

Figure 5.1 Matrix generated by Macrepertory using expert analysis setting.

Management

Polybowel nosode (Helios) 30C 1 pill daily 3 days then Aqua Sanicula LM1 in 10% alcohol, 30ml, 2 drops daily in water with 10 succussions before each dose.

Ipecac 30C if required for nausea and Nitric acid 30C if required for mouth ulcers.

Nutritional supplements: cod liver oil, Selenium with vitamins C and E, and B multivitamins.

I usually advise waiting 2 weeks after a bowel nosode before beginning a fundamental remedy, but her illness and her treatment are moving quickly and her vitality is good. Helios Polybowel nosode consists of Bach's bowel nosodes – Morgan Co and Dysentery Co and Gaertneer and Proteus plus Paterson's Sycotic Co, mixed in equal parts at 9C then potentised up to 30C using 40 hand succussions at each step.

Consultation 14th April 2005

She lost a little weight but she's so much happier in herself. It is now 4 weeks since her surgery to remove the tumour. She was only in hospital for 5 days after the operation and they thought she would need to be in for 10 days. And then she had the last of the intensive chemotherapy courses and this time, for the first time ever, she did not need hospital admission with fever and sore mouth, because she didn't get either the fever or the sore mouth or the bowel infection.

So I've not had to give her the nitric acid. The Ipecec didn't work for the nausea so I soon stopped it. Since the surgery she has lost one kg but some of that was probably the weight of the tumour.

Her appetite has been OK these last 2 weeks and she is a lot more vigorous and has a better attitude. The constipation is less and softer but still rabbit droppings.

At surgery the mass was attached to the iliac artery and down into the pelvis and fixed to the left fallopian tube so they removed the tube but left the ovary. The tumour just peeled away easily from the iliac vessels and the surgeon felt that it was not attached. They could not find the secondary in the right side of her pelvis found on the scans, which was the size of a mandarin orange and they have no explanation. The tumour was 90% dead. It was the size of a grapefruit and at the core the living part was trying to make a kidney. Her wound healed so well and so fast.

She is much brighter and better emotionally. She is much stronger in herself. She is like my daughter again.

She is facing another eight 3 week cycles of less intensive chemo-therapy plus 5 weeks of 5 cycles of 5 days of radiotherapy which might be electron stream therapy and not heavy radiation. I am going to talk to the radiotherapist as I really don't want her to have powerful radiotherapy as it is likely to damage her pelvic and femoral growth.

At the surgery they put in a plastic bag which they can fill with saline to lift the abdominal contents out of the way when they do the radiotherapy.

Her eyelashes have started growing.

Management

Patient advised to continue Aqua Sanicula LM1 2 drops daily till finished then begin LM3 drops daily till all conventional treatment is over.

Outcome

She had the milder chemotherapy cycles without significant problems and then electron beam therapy without any problems. Her hair grew back rapidly and she became well and happy.

CASE 5.2 Recurrent otitis media with perforation and glue ear

Context

R is a 3-year-old girl with curly blonde hair and blue-green eyes – tall and very thin.

Consultation November 2003

R had febrile convulsions at 6 months and then started with otitis media from 10 months. By 11 months old she had grommets. From 1 year old she has always had ear infections one after the other and had more operations for grommets for glue ears. In August she was admitted to hospital with suspected encephalitis. I'm here because the E.N.T. specialist has suggested long term antibiotics and I don't want that. She's already had so many antibiotics since she was 10 months old. She's had a cough for the last month and is coughing up a load of mucous.

She's not a good eater and is getting very thin. She's on the 97th centile for height, but only the 50th centile for weight. Yes, she was breast fed for 11 months. She won't eat warm or cold food, everything has to be tepid. She wants dry food, like crisp-bread and carrots in separate bowls. She gets stomach ache when she eats, more after milk in the morning. Her bowels are very loose. She is always drinking and is always very thirsty.

Her ears run all the time, especially the left and her balance is not good. She is worse if she is too hot and is always stripping of her clothes. She wakes at night and sleeps on top of the covers.

She throws herself on the floor and ignores me when she is upset. But she needs so much attention. She always needs me to be interacting with her. When she is well, she can be happy and helpful and chatty and friendly.

I've found that Chamomilla really helps her when she is teething and it helps her moodiness a bit and sometimes it helps when she wakes from sleep crying and cries for an hour. No, it does not help her ear infections. My husband's family are all doctors in South Africa and they are all against Homeopathy.

She had B.C.G. vaccine 12 hours after birth because that is the fashion in South Africa. She had measles at 18 months. Her other immunisations were at the usual times and she was OK. She had the HIB booster 6 weeks ago.

Observation: R is very restless, never stops moving. She whines a lot and keeps interrupting her mother and needs mum to interact with her a lot. She plays by herself only for a short while, then is upset again and needs mum.

The first otitis media was bilateral but the last 4 have been the left side. When she has an ear infection the ears discharges lots of yellow-green pus constantly and it stinks – like rotten decaying fish and she has a slight fever, but not much. In between ear infections her ears discharge lots of wax and it stinks – like sour milk, or like compost. The left ear has been running with lots of wax for 8 weeks now.

The cough this month is of clear mucous, worse at night, worse from excitement, worse after lying down for a while. She coughs it out when she sits up.

She says she gets stomach ache with most foods. She hates sloppy wet food and soup. She hates anything new. She loves raw vegetables, especially raw carrots; plain boiled white rice and plain boiled pasta. She adores fruit.

She has a slump in energy between 11 and 12 and after nursery at 3.30 and from 7 p.m. She is best after lunch. She is a thumb sucker and has a comfort blanket. After a sleep during the day she wakes up super-charged and raring to go.

The pregnancy was wonderful – I didn't even have any nausea. I broke my ankle at 6 months. I played golf 3 times a week and I never felt so well. Yes, she is my first child. Yes, she is my first conception.

We moved here after my husband's business collapsed and he had a nervous breakdown and I've been very ill. If I cry R comforts me but she gets very distressed.

There is a lot of cancer in the family – her maternal grandfather and both paternal grandparents.

She hates the wind blowing in her ears and cries and puts her hands over her ears. She is hot like her father and has more energy in the evening and after a snooze. She was fine when we were skiing in Sweden and it was minus 32 degrees. She is very restless in her sleep – she is like an electric eel.

She is very busy and restless and can't settle to play. She has temper tantrums – she lies on the floor screaming and kicking and waving her arms. She is very touchy and cuddly – she was never put down when she was little. She needs to be carried or rocked all the time when she is ill – it's been like that since her first illness – it's the only thing that will quiet her.

On examination: lots of smelly wax both sides, tympanic membranes not red, healed central perforation on left tympanic membrane. No grommets seen.

Analysis

Symptoms suggestive of Chamomilla:

• Amelioration of teething and moodiness by Chamomilla.
• Amelioration from being carried quickly.
• Desire for being rocked and amelioration from rocking.

Yet Chamomilla does not help the otitis media or smelly discharges from the ears. Another medicine is required which will act as "the chronic of Chamomilla".

She's had so many courses of antibiotics so is very likely to have altered her bowel flora and she is immune suppressed and so needs a bowel nosode.

Rubrics

• Chronic in the same sentence as chamomilla (9)*: *acon.*, **Aq-Sanic.**, *coff.*, con., **Grat.**, hell., mag-m., puls., staph.
• Fish Brine Odours (15)**: **AQ-SANIC.**, ba-tn., **Calc.**, choc., cimic., falco-p., hydrog., lappa, **Med.**, ozone, pitu-a., sabin., sep., syc-co., thuj.
• Rocked, desires to be (10).*
• Rocking; ameliorates (22).*
• Ears; inflammation; middle ear.
• Ears; perforation, tympanum (22).
• Ears; suppuration; middle ear.
• Ears; Eustachian tubes.

In 2003 MacRepertory analysis gave Chamomilla as the 1st remedy and Aqua Sanicula as the 3rd. Retrospective analysis using Complete Repertory 2015 using the same rubrics (Figure 5.2) gives Aqua Sanicula as the 1st remedy and Chamomilla as the 5th.

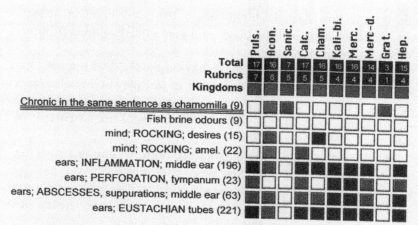

Figure 5.2 Matrix generated by Macrepertory using expert analysis setting.

Management

PolyBowel Nosode 30CH, 3 doses, 12 hours apart. Two weeks later Aqua Sanicula LM1 in 10% alcohol, 30ml teat bottle, 2 drops daily in water with 10 succussions before each dose.

Consultation January 2004

There was no change after the bowel nosode for a week and then her stomach ache just disappeared and has not come back. Her stools went pale. Her bowels have been moving every day and the constipation and diarrhoea are gone. She is eating better.

Then at 2 weeks she had a massive ear infection. She had pain in her right ear and fever for 24 hours, then her eardrum burst and she started pouring out a huge amount of foul-smelling pus. It really stank. After a week of the pus I took her to get antibiotics.

I interrupt with one clear strong word – "Good" and Mum smiles and carries straight on with – but for the first time ever I did not need to finish the bottle.

She was having offensive discharges from all the outlets of her body – her nose, her vomit and some diarrhoea. After a week the pus stopped and her perforation healed. Her body purged itself and it was good.

At 4 weeks we moved house and we all love it. She is sleeping better – I just put her in bed and she goes to sleep quickly – it is wonderful.

My mother became seriously ill on the 27th December and was rushed to hospital. She nearly died and I've been really worried since.

She is home now. Rachel is highly strung, like me. When I am irritable then so is she and then she plays on it and winds me up even more. When I'm relaxed, Rachel is relaxed.

She is calmer, happier and much less clingy. She does not need me to interact with her all the time – she can just play by herself. She is hearing better. She has had no time off nursery school even with the ear infection. Everyone has said what a wonderful change there is in her.

She still gets a bit hyperactive for a few hours if Grandma gives her sweets or lemonade or a Big Mac when they are out.

The wax is back to normal now and no smell. Her breath is normal – the stink has gone. Her tongue is no longer coated and she has put on some weight. She has lots of good happy energy.

Since my mother has been so ill, I've forgotten to give the drops. She's not had any for about 10 days and I think she's beginning to slip back a bit in her mood, but she is still so much better than before. Her body seems to be self-regulating now.

Management

Re-start Aqua Sanicula LM1 drops daily till end of bottle or until mum just forgets to give it. Order Aqua Sanicula LM3 and keep it till next acute otitis media or other acute illness. Advised to return for review during next otitis but she has remained well.

Related Remedies

Share and Compare at level of Clinical Rubric Clusters

- Prolapse of uterus – actual or sensation as if.
- Sepia officinalis and Murex purpurea and Carbo animalis and Lappa arcticum.

- Odour of fish or rotting cheese from orifices.
- Tellurium, Thuja occidentalis, Medorrhinum, Hepar sulph, Oleum animale and Psorinum.

- Constipation – huge, receding or square stool – impaction with overflow.
- Silicea terra, Natrum muriaticum and Opium.

- Anxiety and fear from downward motion.
- Borax and Gelsemium sempervirens.

Other Aqua – related at the Sensation Level plus Clinical Rubric Clusters

Aqua Skookum Chuck, Aqua Marina, Aqua Teplitz, Aqua Hochstein, Aqua Carlsbad, Aqua Kissingen and Aqua Vichy Grande Grille.

- DELUSIONS, imaginations; Gave way; everything under him (5): aq-sanic., aq-tep., cypra-e., digin., kali-br.
- KICKS; child is cross, kicks and scolds (11): aq-hoch., **Aq-Sanic.**, bufo, **CHAM.**, cina, cupr., kreos., **Lyc.**, *plut-n.*, psor., scorp.

Eyes

- INFLAMMATION; bathing, washing; ameliorates, cold (6): **Apis**, aq-mar., aq-sanic., asar., puls., **Syph**.

Throat

- GREY (8): aq-hoch., aq-sanic., **Iod.**, **Kali-m.**, lyc., **Merc-cy.**, phel., **Phyt.**
- PAIN; sore, bruised; uvula (13): am-m., aq-carl., aq-sanic., calc., canth., caust., chlor., nat-ar., nit-ac., ptel., ruta, sabin., **Sang**.

Rectum

- URGING, desire; flatus; aggravates (9): **ALOE**, **Aq-Sanic.**, aq-vichy-g., hedeo., nat-s., **Nux-v.**, oxyg., ruta, spig.

Extremities

- EXCORIATION; feet; soles (11): **Aq-Sanic.**, **Aq-Skook.**, **Bar-c.**, **Calc.**, **Graph.**, **NIT-AC.**, nux-v., petr., sabad., sep., **SIL.**

Chill

- POSTPONING, belated (12): alst-s., aq-kiss., aq-sanic., bry., *canth.*, chin., cina, **GAMB.**, ign., **Ip.**, kali-bi., phos.

Carbons

Remedies: Graphites and Petroleum and Carbo animalis.

Skin

- Cracks, crusts and scabs, full of, hands (4): **Anthr.**, **Aq-Sanic.**, **GRAPH.**, **Petr.**

Face

- SADDLE across nose (10): aq-sanic., **Carb-an.**, chel., ictod., lyc., op., **SEP.**, sulph., syph., tril.

Asteraceae

Remedies: Chamomilla, Gnaphallium polycephalum, Lappa arcticum.

Chamomilla

- CAPRICIOUSNESS; children, in (10): aq-sanic., **CHAM.**, **CINA**, Nux-v., op., plac., **Puls.**, rheum, sac-alb., staph.
- ROCKING; desires (15): Acon., aq-sanic., **Carb-an.**, **CHAM.**, Cina, coloc., dpt, herin., kali-c., merc-c., puls., pyrog., rhus-t., stram., verat.

Gnaphallium polycephalum

- Stomach; APPETITE; wanting; children, babies, in (12): alum., aq-sanic., bar-c., calc., cina, **Gnaph.**, lac-d., lac-h., lyc., nat-p., sac-alb., tub.
- Rectum; DIARRHOEA; summer; children, in (19): apoc., **Aq-Sanic.**, **Bell.**, **Calc.**, **Calc-p.**, **Cham.**, cuph., epil., **Ferr.**, **Ferr-p.**, **Gnaph.**, ip., **Iris**, **Psor.**, sec., thuj., typh., **Verat.**, **Zinc.**

Lappa arcticum

Female

- PROLAPSE; uterus; standing; aggravates (4): aq-sanic., **Lappa**, nit-ac., **Sep.**

Energy Remedies: X Ray, Electricitas, Magnetus polus arcticus

Face

- PAIN; dull; jaws; upper (3): aq-sanic., lob-c., x-ray.

Back

- GOOSE flesh (6): aq-sanic., calc-ar., carc., electr., plut-n., **Sarr.**

Chest

- OPPRESSION; sudden, paroxysmal (9): aq-sanic., carb-v., cina, *kreos.*, *lach.*, *m-arct.*, **Mag-m.**, plb., plb-acet.

Birds

Remedies: Peregrine Falcon and Bald Eagle.

- FORGETFULNESS; Details, for (3): aq-sanic., cadm., falco-p.

Back

- COLDNESS, chilliness; wet cloth, as from; sacral region (2): aq-sanic., haliae-lc.

Sarcodes

Remedies: Placenta humana, DNA, Pituitary- anterior, Cortisone, Moschus.

- CONCENTRATION; difficult; one subject, on (8): aq-sanic., hyosin., lac-lup., lsd, *plac.*, plect., senec., tab.

Back

- PAIN; lumbar region, lumbago; lying; ameliorates; side, on (4): aq-sanic., des-ac., nat-s., zinc.

Extremities

- PAIN; sore, bruised; hands; left (3): aq-sanic., pitu-a., succ.

Generalities

- PAIN; joints, articulations; lying; ameliorates (6): aq-sanic., cortiso., diph., merc-i-r., puls., term-a.

Head

- COLDNESS, chilliness; damp, wet sensation (3): aq-sanic., mosch., thea.

Gemstones

Remedies: Diamond, Emerald, Amethyst.

Head

- PAIN, headache; Forehead; left; extending to; ear (4): adam., aq-sanic., clad-r., maland.

Face

- ERUPTIONS; itching; chin; beard (4): aq-sanic., croto-t., lap-be-e., sars.
- DELUSIONS, imaginations; walk, walking; someone walks; behind him (11): *amet.*, anac., aq-sanic., **Calc.**, crot-c., diox., ferr., mag-m., med., mur-ac., **Staph.**

Nosodes

Remedies: Tuberculinum bovinum, Variolinum, Sycotic Co., Dysentery Co., Medorrhinum, Bacillinum.

- OCCUPATION, diversion; changing his, constantly (4): **Apis, Aq-Sanic.,** bor., tub.

Head

- CRAZY feeling (3): aq-sanic., lil-t., vario.
- PERSPIRATION; profuse; night (5): aq-sanic., calc., camph., sulph., **Syc-co.**

Stomach

- FULLNESS; loosen clothing, must (2): aq-sanic., dys-co.

Extremities

- PAIN; feet; soles; uncover, inclination to (7): **AQ-SANIC.**, **Cham.**, helo., **Lach.**, **Med.**, **Sang.**, **Sulph.**

Rectum

- INACTIVITY; chronic (4): alum., aq-sanic., bac., sep.

Gases

Remedies: Nitrous oxide, Neon, Hydrogen and Ozone.

- DELUSIONS, imaginations; Seasick, that he is (6): aq-sanic., der., lar-ar., magn-gr., nitro-o., tab.

Extremities

- PAIN; shoulders; right; extending to; neck (3): aq-sanic., neon, sac-l.

Back

- PAIN; lying; side, on, ameliorates (15): aq-sanic., cist., des-ac., hydrc., hydrog., *irid.*, kali-n., *nat-c.*, nat-s., nicc-s., nux-v., **Puls.**, tama., ust., zinc.

Mouth

- APHTHAE; white (14): aq-sanic., **Ars.**, **Bor.**, brucel., **Cic.**, **Hell.**, kali-chl., methylp-h., **Nit-ac.**, ozone, sal-ac., sin-a., **Sul-ac.**, toxop-p.

Milks

Remedies: Lac caninum, Lac vaccinum defloratum and Lac equinum.

Head; PAIN, headache;

- Stitching; Occiput; right; extending to:
- Forehead (10): aq-sanic., bar-c., bov., chel., ferr-p., **LAC-C.**, nat-m., ozone, sars., thuj.

Generalities

CLOTHING; sensation of; damp, wet (13): aq-sanic., *calc.*, cassi-f., guai., **Lac-d.**, lyc., phos., **Ran-b.**, rhod., sapin., sep., tub., verat-v.

- ANGER: touch aggravates (9): **Ant-c.**, **Aq-Sanic.**, cham., **Cina**, falco-p., **Iod.**, lac-eq., lach., **TARENT.**

Aethusa cynapium

Stomach

- VOMITING; milk; gushing (3): aq-sanic., **Aeth.**, carc.
- VOMITING; milk; after; mother's; nursing, directly after (5): **AETH.**, **Ant-c.**, aq-sanic., ip., **Sil.**
- VOMITING; milk; curdled; lumps, large (5): **Aeth.**, aq-sanic., calc., past., **Valer.**
- VOMITING; projectile (12): acon., *aeth.*, apom., aq-sanic., **BELL.**, *cupr.*, dys-co., op., phos., thyr., **VERAT.**, verat-v.

> This symptom requires urgent admission to hospital for investigation. Baby may have pyloric stenosis and require surgery.

- VOMITING; sleep; before (8): **Aeth.**, ant-t., aq-sanic., bell., croto-t., **Cupr.**, cycl., **Nat-m.**

Sleep

- FALLING asleep; vomiting, after (6): **Aeth.**, ant-t., aq-sanic., bell., cupr., nat-m.
- SLEEPINESS; vomiting; after (17): **Aeth.**, ant-c., **ANT-T.**, apoc., **Apom.**, **Aq-Sanic.**, ars., *bell.*, chin-ar., cupr., cycl., dig., **IP.**, kali-bi, strep-s., verat., vip.

References

1   Clarke, JH. *Dictionary of Practical Materia Medica* Vol 2 (3rd edn). Sittingbourne Kent: Homeopathic Book Service, 1991. pp. 1090–1102.
2   Van Zandvoot, R. *Complete Repertory*. Leidschendam, NL: Institute for Research in Homeopathic Information and Symptomatology, 1996. (Accessed via MacRepertory version 8.0.)

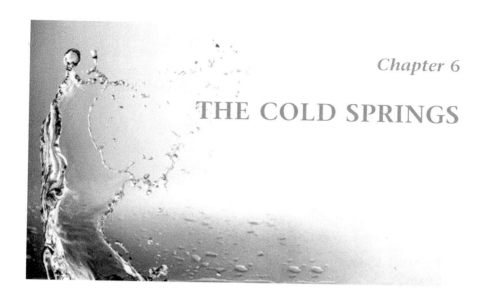

Chapter 6

THE COLD SPRINGS

The Cold Springs included in this book are:

Aqua Adelheid, Aqua Bartfelder, Aqua Bondonneau, Aqua Ems, Aqua Franzensbad, Aqua Friedrichshaller, Aqua Gettysburg, Aqua Hall, Aqua Hochstein, Aqua Jatzfeld, Aqua Kissingen, Aqua Kronthal, Aqua Landeck, Aqua Lippspringe, Aqua Meinberg Pyrmont, Aqua Tunbridge Wells, Aqua Vichy Hospital, Aqua Voeslau, Aqua Weilbach, Aqua Wiesbaden, Aqua Wildbad.

AQUA ADELHEID

Source

A cold mineral spring rising at Adelheid, Heilbrunn, in Bavaria, Germany, mentioned by A. Albright in the American Journal of Pharmacy 1835–1907 in the September 1859 edition on page 458 with the contents of the spring. There is no proving: symptoms from drinking the water, bathing in spa and cured cases.

Contents

- Row 2: carbonic acid, dissolved oxygen and nitrogen gases.
- Row 3: Sodium bromate, sodium carbonate, sodium iodate, sodium sulphate, magnesium carbonate, aluminium oxide, silica.
- Row 4: Ferrous carbonate.

Rubrics[1]

Sensitivity and vulnerability: emotional and cognitive – loss of resilience – overwhelm

- SING, desires to; thrilling (13): acon., aq-adel., BELL., Cocc., lyc., mag-c., nat-c., nux-v., phos., staph., stram., ther., verat.
- TOSSING about; night; bed, in (11): abies-c., acon., aq-adel., calc., Cham., mag-c., nat-m., nux-v., petr., phos., sabad.
- RESTLESSNESS, nervousness; night; bed, in (19): abies-c., acon., aq-adel., ars., calc., Caust., Cham., graph., mag-c., mag-m., merc., nat-m., nux-v., petr., phos., rauw., ros-g., sabad., sid-al.

Abdomen

- RUMBLING noise; coffee ameliorates (3): aq-adel., aq-carl., phos.

Generalities

- FOOD drinks; fried food, aversion to (3): aq-adel., mag-s., Plb.
- FOOD drinks; roasted food, aversion to (5): aq-adel., agar., mand., ptel., tarent.
- FOOD drinks; fruits; desires; sour, acid (25): acal., *adon.*, Ant-t., aq-adel., Ars., bufo, calc., calc-s., chin., Cist., cub., cypra-e., euon-a., *hep.*, hyosin., ign., lach., Mag-c., Med., nabal., Phos., ptel., *ther.*, thuj., VERAT.

Clinical rubrics

Skin

- Boils – small multiple recurrent with enlarged adjacent lymph nodes.
- Hard pimples with a red inflamed areola, itching somewhat with a yellow, pustular apex, somewhat moist on scratching it off (like small boils), on neck, chest, fingers and toes.
- Small, hard indurations in the palm of the hand, very near the last joint of the fourth finger, adherent to the bone.

Thyroid goitre and Epistaxis – recurrent

Food and drinks

• Desires: sour, acid food fruit; potatoes and other vegetables.

Compare Related Remedy

Aqua Carlsbad

Abdomen

• RUMBLING noise: coffee ameliorates (3): aq-adel., aq-carl., phos.

AQUA BARTFELDER

Source

A cold acid spring rising at Bardejov Kupele in Slovakia near the Polish border

Contents

• Row 3: sodium carbonate, sodium chloride and silica.
• Row 4: potassium carbonate, potassium chloride and ferrous carbonate.

Rubrics

Sensitivity and vulnerability – emotional and cognitive – loss of resilience – overwhelm

• SLEEPINESS; coffee, after (2): aq-bart., lach.
• ANXIETY; coffee; aggravates (5): aq-bart., **CHAM.**, *ign.*, **Nux-v.**, stram.

Stomach

• APPETITE; increased, hunger in general; morning; breakfast, after (4): aloe, aq-bart., **Sulph.**, tax.

Suppression of emotions – Sublimation of libido

Generalities

• Swarming sensation on body (1): aq-bart.

Eyes

- PAIN; coition, after (3): aq-bart., **Cedr.**, nat-m.

Female

- COITION; enjoyment; diminished (6): aq-bart., caul., ferr-p., plat., sep., tarent.
- COITION; aversion to, sexual aversion; menses; after (9): aq-bart., arund., berb., **Caust.**, kali-c., *nat-m.*, **Phos.**, sep., *sul-ac.*

Male

- COITION; enjoyment; diminished (5): aq-bart., phos., plat., sep., tarent.

Water

Female

- PAIN; burning, smarting; bathing, washing aggravates (1): aq-bart.
- PAIN; bathing, washing; aggravates (3): aq-bart., crot-c., eupi.

Urethra

- PAIN; twinging; meatus; bathing, washing aggravates (1): aq-bart.

Clinical Rubric Clusters

Achilles Tendons

- Especially left – contracture, spasms, numbness, pulsation.

Extremities

- CONTRACTION; muscles, tendons; convulsive, spasmodic; calves (4): aq-bart., ars., merc., sil.
- NUMBNESS, insensibility; legs; tendo achilles; left (1): aq-bart.
- NUMBNESS, insensibility; legs; tendo achilles (2): aq-bart., hell.
- PULSATION; legs; tendo achilles; left (2): aq-bart., prun.
- PULSATION; legs; tendo achilles (3): aq-bart., prun., zinc.

Skin – Corns, Boils Urticaria

Extremities

- CORNS; stitching, stinging; night; bed, in (3): aq-bart., rhod., **Sulph.**
- CORNS; stitching, stinging; night (5): aq-bart., ars., nat-m., rhod., **Sulph.**

Skin

- ERUPTIONS; urticaria, nettle-rash; morning (4): aq-bart., **Bell.**, bov., chin.
- ERUPTIONS; urticaria, nettle-rash; evening (9): aq-bart., hyper., *indg.*, **Kreos.**, lyc., **Nux-v.**, oxpr., tarent-c., titan.

Abdomen

- ERUPTIONS; pustules; evening (1): aq-bart.
- ERUPTIONS; pustules (17): **Ant-c.**, ant-o., **Ant-t.**, apis, aq-bart., chlol., clem., crot-c., croto-t., kali-bi., merc., nat-m., puls., sep., squil., toxop-p., tub.

Haemorrhoids – formicating, painful, strangulated

Rectum

- HAEMORRHOIDS; strangulated, irreducible (21): acon., **Aesc.**, **ALOE**, aq-bart., ars., **Bell.**, **Canth.**, **Caps.**, colch., **Coloc.**, **Ign.**, **LACH.**, lob., **Merc.**, mez., **Nux-v.**, **PAEON.**, rat., sep., **Sil.**, **Sulph.**
- HAEMORRHOIDS: burning, smarting (104); formicating, crawling (30); painful (185); protruding, prolapsed (92)

Useful or Unusual Rubrics

Sleep

- YAWNING; walking; while (8): aq-bart., camph., chlf., eug., euphr., kali-c., lycps., stann.

Abdomen

- PAIN; drawing; gripping; morning, on waking (1): aq-bart.
- PAIN; drawing; gripping (5): aq-bart., asaf., dios., hyos., phos.

Urethra

- PAIN; meatus; bathing, washing aggravates (1): aq-bart.
- PAIN; twinging; meatus; bathing, washing aggravates (1): aq-bart.
- PAIN; twinging; meatus (3): aq-bart., berb., zinc.
- PAIN; twinging (9): aq-bart., arg-n., **Berb.**, **Cann-s.**, carb-v., clem., lyc., **Sel.**, zinc.

Heart and circulation

- Palpitation heart; coffee, after (23).

Back

- LAMENESS; lumbar region; evening (1): aq-bart.
- PAIN; paralytic; lumbar region; evening (3): alum., aq-bart., **Kalm.**

Compare/related remedies

Chamomilla and Nux vomica

- ANXIETY; coffee; aggravates (5): aq-bart., **CHAM.**, *ign.*, **Nux-v.**, stram.

Generalities

- COFFEE; aggravates (24): **All-c.**, ang., aq-bart., arg., arg-n., calc., calc-p., **CHAM.**, chlor., eug., fl-ac., *ign.*, **Lach.**, mill., mobil-ph., nat-m., **Nux-v.**, osm., ph-ac., phos., stram., **Sul-ac.**, **Thuj.**, tub.

Skin

- ERUPTIONS; urticaria, nettle-rash; evening (9): aq-bart., hyper., *indg.*, **Kreos.**, lyc., **Nux-v.**, oxpr., tarent-c., titan.

Energy remedies

Abdomen

- PAIN; drawing; morning (8): aq-bart., **Calc.**, con., **M-arct.**, mang-acet., merc-i-r., nat-c., phos.

AQUA BONDONNEAU

Source

Water from the cold effervescent chalybeate springs at Bondonneau near Montelimar in southeast France.

History

Roman baths from 100 B.C. – Napoleon III re-opened the spa in 1857 but never as popular as the hot spas.

Contents

- Row 2: carbonic acid.
- Row 3: sodium bicarbonate, sodium chloride, sodium sulphate, magnesium carbonate, magnesium sulphate, alumina, silica sulphuric acid.
- Row 4: potassium sulphate, ferrous oxide, manganese oxide, traces of arsenic and bromides.
- Row 5: trace of iodine.

Rubrics

Sensitivity and vulnerability: emotional and cognitive – loss of resilience – overwhelm

- Excitable excitement aggravates.
- Anxiety – painful anxiety, anguish.
- Startling – on falling asleep from sleep.
- Sleeplessness after excitement.
- Dreams – many interrupts sleep.
- Sleepy during the day.
- Tension throughout the body – Grinding teeth at night – tension fullness around the heart – tumultuous palpitations worse after eating.
- Irritability anger.
- Whole skin surface feels oversensitive to touch temperature.

Suppression of emotions – Sublimation of libido

- Persistent sexual thoughts.
- Sensation as if heat/or dryness in vagina.
- Sensation as if heat fullness in the chest.
- Paroxysms of spasmodic oppression of chest, with hiccough.
- Frequent morning erections.
- Hardness of the breasts.

Desire to Beget Children be a Parent

- Sensation as if of oppression of chest with sensation of head of foetus abutting under the sternum.

Sensations *as if*

- Teeth are too long.
- Increased sensitivity of whole skin surface to touch temperature with itching tickling prickling.
- Heaviness: whole body, head.
- Compression of eyeballs.
- Tension swelling drawing in eyelids.
- Swelling of the tonsils heat prickling in tonsils.

Generalities

- Induration swelling: lymphatic tissue, spleen, liver, breasts.
- Pains: shooting, darting, lightning, quick, cutting, sore, bruised.
- Dryness mucous membranes.
- Emaciation even cachexia despite increased appetite hunger.

- Discharges secretions: profuse, thin, liquid, green with swellings stitching pains.
- Morning aggravates swollen sensation of eyelids.
- Evening aggravates: pallor of conjunctivae, mouth face, chilliness, gurgling in stomach teeth feel too long.
- Eating aggravates burning heat in stomach, tumultuous action of the heart, pain in kidneys.

Head

- Sensation of heaviness.
- Internal pulsation at base of brain – worse in evening.
- Congestive compressive throbbing headache with prickling in throat or drawing itching of scalp – worse moving head.
- Swelling of temporal veins throbbing in veins – veins not tender – associated with swollen veins of hands.
- Sensation of constriction in forehead with irascibility.
- Vertigo with dim vision.

Eyes

- Red painless swelling of lachrymal ducts.
- Lancinating pains in orbits with evening chilliness.
- Itching lids photophobia.
- Yellow sclera pale conjunctiva.

Throat

- Tonsillitis with bright red throat swollen lymph nodes.

Chest

- Bronchitis – acute, recurrent chronic inflammation of bronchi.

Spine and Extremities

- Drawing stiffness in the cervical muscles.
- Constant heat in the palms of the hands.
- Stiffness sensitiveness of the finger-joints.

Skin

- Pimples: sensitive, colourless itching appear in succession, on the face.
- Ulcers: skin ulcers cease suppurating while taking the water for a long while after, with general improvement of the health – even profusely suppurating fistulous ulcers on the tibia leave off suppurating.

Male

- Serous or mucous discharge from prepuce with itching.

Useful or Unusual Rubrics

Throat

- HEAT; tonsils (2): aq-bond., iris.
- PAIN; lancinating; tonsils (9): **Amyg-am.**, aq-bond., chel., cub., **Hep.**, merc-i-f., ran-s., raph., ust.

Chest

- HEAT; sternum; behind (10): ant-t., aq-bond., arum-i., *cast.*, cinnb., kali-n., lach., **Phos.**, **Sang.**, **Sanguin-n.**

Compare/Related Remedies

Nitric acid, Solidago virgaurea.

Related level: Clinical Rubric Clusters

Nitric acid

Male

- MOISTURE; mucous (2): aq-bond., nit-ac.
- MOISTURE; prepuce (10): aq-bond., calc., lach., merc., *nit-ac.*, sep., staph., sulph., sumb., zinc.

Solidago virgaurea

- PAIN; cutting; region of (15): aids, aq-bond., chel., coc-c., germ., **Ipom.**, menth-pu., myric., plb., sapin., scut., solid., **Staph.**, tarent-c., zinc.
- PAIN; extending; bladder, to (26): aq-bond., arg-n., ars., aur., bell., **BERB.**, **Canth.**, chel., coc-c., cupr-acet., ery-a., hedeo., kali-bi., kali-i., **Lac-d.**, lach., **Lyc.**, nit-ac., nux-v., oci., op., petr., phyt., **Sars.**, **Solid.**, tab.

AQUA EAUX BONNES

Source

A cold sulphur spring in France.

Contents

- Row 3: Sodium chloride, magnesium chloride, magnesium sulphate, silica.

- Row 4: Potassium chloride, calcium carbonate, calcium sulphate, and ferrous sulphate.

Rubrics

Sensitivity and vulnerability: emotional and cognitive – loss of resilience – overwhelm

- Rapid perception reasoning – apparent increased mental strength but little resilience leads to restlessness, overwhelm and exhaustion.

Abdomen

- RUMBLING noise; Breakfast; before (3): aq-eaux, *gnaph.*, nat-s.

AQUA EMS

Source

The spring water of the spa town Bad Ems in Rhineland-Palatinate in Germany.

Contents

No analysis of contents can be found. The town of Bad Ems still exists but no longer as a spa.

Rubrics

Clinical Rubric Clusters – Salivation and Pancreas

Salivation

Generalities

- STIFFNESS, rigidity; salivation, from suppressed (1): aq-ems.
- SALIVATION ameliorates (5): acon., aq-ems, brom., sul-ac., thuj.

Mouth

- SALIVATION; pain, during; abdomen, left (1): aq-ems.

- SALIVATION; pain, during; abdomen (5): aq-ems, *gran.*, *kali-c.*, *sulph.*, *zinc.*
- SALIVATION; suppressed (10): aq-ems, bell., cahin., cann-s., kali-br., merc-c., op., phyt., stram., trif-r.

Stomach

- RETCHING, gagging; salivation, with (7): *ant-t.*, aq-ems, *calc.*, *croto-t.*, hep., **Lob.**, **Nat-c.**

Rectum

- DIARRHOEA: salivation, from suppressed (1): aq-ems.

Perspiration

- SOUR odour; salivation, from suppressed (1): aq-ems.

Pancreas – pain and inflammation

Abdomen

- SWELLING; pancreas (1): aq-ems
- HARDNESS; pancreas (6): aq-ems, bar-m., but-ac., **Carb-an.**, merc-cy., stry.
- PAIN; pancreas; salivation, from suppressed (1): aq-ems
- PAIN; pancreas (15): aesc-g., aq-ems, ars., **Calc-ar.**, colch., **Iris**, kali-bi., *merc.*, merc-i-r., phos., plat., plb., psor., rhus-t., stann.
- SWELLING; sides; left (4): aq-ems, *calc.*, cean., led.
- SWELLING; sides (8): aq-ems, bry., calc., cean., laur., led., **Rhus-t.**, tub.

Heart and circulation

- PAIN; boring, heart region (9): aq-ems, aur., aur-m., **Cupr.**, mag-p., rhod., **Seneg.**, sep., still.

AQUA FRANZENSBAD

Source

The cold sparkling alkaline-saline spring rising at the spa town of Frantiskovy Lazne in the Czech Republic.

Contents

The water has a high concentration of dissolved carbon dioxide.

- Row 2: Carbon dioxide and carbonic acid.
- Row 3: Sodium chloride and magnesium chloride.
- Row 4: Potassium chloride and calcium chloride.

Rubrics

Sensitivity and vulnerability: emotional and cognitive – loss of resilience – overwhelm

- ANXIETY; afternoon; aggravates; colic, in (1): aq-franz.

Face

- CONTRACTION; sensation of; eyebrows; between (1): aq-franz.
- FROWNING; sensation (3): adam., aq-franz., *enal-c.*
- FROWNING (9): adam., alum., aq-franz., enal-c., hell., mangi., merc-c., *stram.*, zinc.
- CONTRACTION; sensation of (16).

Throat

- CHOKING, constricting; supper ameliorates (1): aq-franz.
- CHOKING, constricting; nausea; with (4): aq-franz., *gent-c.*, kali-cy., *meny.*

Suppression of emotion – Sublimation of Libido

Throat

- CONSTRICTION, closure, contraction; forenoon (2): aq-franz., **Calc.**

Rectum

- JERKING (8): aq-franz., bell., bry., chin., nux-v., rumx., **Sil.**, zinc.

Male

- TINGLING, prickling; penis; prepuce (10): aloe, aq-franz., jac., jac-c., merc., ph-ac., seneg., sumb., tarax., thuj.
- SEXUAL, libido; desire; wanting; erections; with (18): **Alum.**, aq-franz., bry., caj., **Calad.**, clem., crot-c., eug., ferr-ma., fl-ac., kali-c., mag-c., nit-ac., nux-v., ped., spig., sulph., tarent.

Exhaustion – mind and body

- WORK; Mental; aversion to; evening (9): aq-franz., calc-p., carb-ac., form., lyss., nat-m., sol-t-ae., spig., sumb.

Head

- SENSITIVENESS; mental exertion agg. (1): aq-franz.

Eyes

- SENSITIVE; mental exertion aggravates (1): aq-franz.
- MENTAL exertion aggravates (9): adam., agar., aq-franz., cina, ign., **Nux-v.**, pic-ac., pter-a., stach.

Generalities

- WEAKNESS; Muscles Walking; while

Clinical Rubric Clusters

Back Pain

Back

- HEAVINESS, weight; lumbar region; turning in bed, on (2): aq-franz., **Corn.**
- PAIN; pinching; dorsal region; scapulae; below right (1): aq-franz.
- PAIN; pressing; morning; rising from lying ameliorates (4): aq-franz., kali-n., nat-m., staph.
- PAIN; pressing; morning; waking, on (10): aq-franz., arg-n., berb., dulc., ign., kali-c., lach., nit-ac., staph., **Zinc.**
- PAIN; chronic; lumbar region (10): aesc., aq-franz., berb., **Calc-f.**, gnaph., lant., **Morg.**, **Rhus-t.**, sil., **Solid.**

Irritable bowel syndrome

Abdomen; PAIN; Sore, bruised

- Pressure; aggravates; hard, firm (3): aq-franz., atro., fago.
- Bed; in; ameliorates (6): aq-franz., **Ars.**, **Coloc.**, sin-n., staph., symph.
- Descending; ameliorates (1): aq-franz.
- Noon, toward, strong pressure aggravates (1): aq-franz.

- Afternoon; three pm; walking aggravates (1): aq-franz.
- Afternoon (9): aq-franz., coloc., fago., lyc., mag-s., nux-v., osm., phyt., **Valer.**
- Evening; seven pm. (7): ammc., aq-franz., elaps, neod., phel., stry., sulph., tela, **Zing.**

- PAIN; stitching; liver region; gallbladder, region of (11): aq-franz., **Aran.**, aran-ix., **Berb.**, dios., **Hep.**, kola., mand., *ran-s.*, *sep.*, thul-p.
- MOVEMENTS; dinner, after (3): aq-franz., **Coloc.**, *ol-an.*

Useful or Unusual Rubrics

Nose

TINGLING, prickling inside

- Nostrils; left (2): aq-franz., lob-s.
- Nostrils (4): aq-franz., lob-s., phys., salx-f.
- Left (10): aq-franz., arg., carb-v., cench., *dros.*, hep., lap-be-e., *leon.*, lob-s., nat-p.

Chest

- PAIN; Extending to; upper limbs; left (5): aq-franz., carc., dys-co., hell., **Kalm.**, lat-m., mangi., spig., tarent.

Compare Related Remedies

Acids

Remedies

Fluoric acid, Picric acid, Phosphoric acid, Nitric acid and Carbolic acid. Related Level = Clinical Rubric Clusters.

Generalities

- PAIN; pressure; aggravates; hard (6): aq-franz., atro., *berb.*, choc., fago., fl-ac.

Back

- HEAVINESS, weight; motion; aggravates (4): aq-franz., **Phos.**, phyt., **Pic-ac.**
- HEAVINESS, weight; morning; bed, in (7): ang., ant-t., aq-franz., euphr., pic-ac., **Sep.**, sulph.
- PAIN; pressing; morning; waking, on (10): aq-franz., arg-n., berb., dulc., ign., kali-c., lach., nit-ac., staph., **Zinc.**

Male

- TINGLING, prickling; penis; prepuce (10): aloe, aq-franz., jac., jac-c., merc., ph-ac., seneg., sumb., tarax., thuj.
- SEXUAL, libido; desire; wanting; erections; with (18): **Alum.**, aq-franz., bry., caj., **Calad.**, clem., crot-c., eug., ferr-ma., fl-ac., kali-c., mag-c., nit-ac., nux-v., ped., spig., sulph., tarent.

- WORK; Mental; aversion to; evening (9): aq-franz., calc-p., carb-ac., form., lyss., nat-m., sol-t-ae., spig., sumb.

AQUA FRIEDRICHSHALLER

Source

Water from the cold spring rising in the district of Heilbronn, Bad Wurtemberg, Germany, also known as Friedrichshaller bitterwasser.

Contents

The analysis of contents of the spring has been lost. The town of Bad Wurtemberg still exists but is not a spa.

Rubrics

Sensitivity and vulnerability: emotional and cognitive – loss of resilience – overwhelm

- EXCITMENT, excitable; ailments from, aggravates.
- HYPOCHONDRIASIS.
- SADNESS and DULLNESS.

- Stomach; APPETITE; increased, hunger in general.
- Male; SEXUAL DESIRE, libido: increased.
- Bladder; URGING to urinate, morbid desire.

Suppression of emotions – Sublimation of libido

- Abdomen; FORMICATION, crawling; umbilical region (7): aq-fried., *caust.*, chel., *grat.*, *paeon.*, plect., **Slag**.
- Generalities; FORMICATION, crawling.
- Sleep: yawning frequent.
- Generalities; tension, tightness.

Water Thirst

Urine

- SCANTY; daytime (4): aesc., aq-fried., **Lyc.**, ther.

Stomach

- THIRST; daytime (19): alum., aq-fried., bell-p., bov., **Bry.**, *cocc.*, con., *hep.*, *kali-n.*, *led.*, methylp-h., naja-m., neon, ol-an., petr., *sars.*, *sulph.*, thuj., zinc.
- THIRST; daytime; drink, with aversion to.

Generalities

- FOOD drinks: drinks; aversion.

Clinical Rubric Clusters

Heartburn and Irritable Bowel Syndrome

Generalities

- PAIN; mucous membranes; burning, smarting.
- FOOD drinks: beer; aggravates.

Stomach

- HEARTBURN.
- PAIN; pressing; drinking aggravates (11): aego-p., ant-t., aq-fried., bruc., chel., **Chin-s.**, *daph.*, hyos., *nux-v.*, ph-ac., sil.
- PAIN: drinking; aggravates; eating; after; eructation; ameliorates.
- PAIN, pressing eating; after; eructation; ameliorates.

Abdomen

- PAIN: hypochondria pressing hypochondria fullness; hypogastrium.

Rectum

- FLATUS: stool; during; urging for stool; flatus is passed, but only; offensive.
- URGING, desire; eating; after diarrhoea.

Stool

- LIQUID, thin.

Beer aggravates

Head

- PAIN, headache; beer; aggravates (16): **ACON.**, *aq-calc-caust.*, aq-fried., bell., calc., caust., **Coc-c.**, coloc., ferr., kali-chl., lappa, merc., methylp-h., nitro., **RHUS-T.**, verat.
- PAIN, headache: evening aggravates stitching.

Generalities

- FOOD drinks: alcohol, alcoholic drinks; aggravate; beer aggravates.
- PAIN: evening aggravates; drinking aggravates; eating; after; eructation ameliorates.
- DISCHARGES, secretions: acid, sour; thin, liquid.
- CONSTRICTION: external FULLNESS: internal.

Bladder

- URINATION; frequent; night. Urine cloudy with sediment.

AQUA GETTYSBURG

Source

An ambient spring in Gettysburg, Pennsylvania, USA – remedy made by trituration of the evaporated water.

Contents

- Row 2: Lithium chloride, nitric acid.
- Row 3: Sodium carbonate, sodium chloride, sodium sulphate, magnesium borate, magnesium carbonate, magnesium sulphate, alumina, silicic acid.
- Row 4: Potassium sulphate, calcium carbonate, calcium fluoride, calcium phosphate, calcium sulphate, ferrous carbonate, cobalt carbonate, niccol carbonate, copper carbonate.
- Row 5: Strontium sulphate.
- Row 6: Barium sulphate.

Rubrics

Sensitivity and vulnerability: emotional and cognitive – loss of resilience – overwhelm

- RESTLESSNESS, nervousness: Midnight; after; one am. (5): aq-get., ars., mang-acet., nat-ar., phos., stann.

Suppression of emotions – Sublimation of libido

Throat

- SWALLOWING; Difficult; Impeded; stiffness of muscles, from (3): aq-get., *arg.*, hyos.

Male

- ATROPHY shrivelled; Penis; bed, in (1): aq-get.

Exhaustion – mental and physical

- WORK; Mental; aversion to:
- Thinking of self, when (1): aq-get.
- Afternoon; busy ameliorates, being (1): aq-get.
- Forenoon (5): alumn., aq-get., fago., lach., pic-ac.
- Afternoon (9): aq-get., bufo-s., hyos., lyc., nat-ar., nat-m., op., pip-m., plan.

Clinical Rubric Clusters

Rheumatic disorders: Polymyalgia rheumatica

Stiffness with palpable rigidity of muscles is the most striking unusual symptom.

Amelioration from rest lying still in bed and aggravation from exertion and motion.

Generalities

- REST; ameliorates; stay long in one position, cannot (1): aq-get.

Extremities

- STIFFNESS, rigidity; lying quietly ameliorates (1): aq-get.
- STIFFNESS, rigidity; morning; motion, on (2): **Apoc.**, aq-get.
- PAIN; rheumatic; rest; ameliorates (6): aq-get., bry., caust., colch., get., mag-p., *squil.*

Osteoarthritis: with sore stiff ligaments after fracture of right piriformis.

Tuberculosis of bone in spine and long bones – as supportive treatment.

Ulcers over bones. Gout.

Extremities

- PAIN; pressing; steel band, as of a narrow, patella, right (1): aq-get.
- PAIN; pressing; knees; patella (8): *acon.*, alum., aq-get., bell., *calc.*, cocc., led., **Sulph.**

- PAIN; rheumatic; tendons (7): aq-get., arn., **Colch.**, form-ac., phyt., rhod., **Rhus-t.**

Chronic fatigue syndrome, ME

- Painful, stiffness and palpable rigidity of muscles.
- Ameliorated by rest – must rest – stay in bed to rest.
- Aggravated by exercise, exertion and motion – feel weak walking, feel weak and faint on walking.
- Aggravated by mental exertion – extremely had to concentrate – even worse thinking of mental work – better just lying-in bed or watching TV.
- Aggravated by thinking: about themselves, about how weak, tired, sore they are all the time.

Catarrh postnasal discharge: clear, frothy, viscid, tough

Nose

- DISCHARGE; Frothy; nares, posterior, choanae (1): aq-get.
- DISCHARGE; Clear; nares, posterior, choanae (8): all-c., aq-get., ars-i., **Kali-m.**, lycpr., nat-m., nat-p., phyll-a.
- DISCHARGE; Viscid, tough; nares, posterior, choanae (38).

Cough with pleuritic pain pleurisy left upper lung

Chest

- PAIN; Upper; left; inspiration aggravates (1): *aq-get.*
- PAIN; Sides; left; inspiration; aggravates (31).**

Cough

- DRY; scraping in; throat, from (4): **Ang.**, **Aq-Get.**, graph., **Sabad.**
- SCRAPING; throat, in (18): am-c., **Ang.**, *aq-get.*, **Arg-n.**, bry., carbn-s., chel., dros., graph., kreos., **Nux-v.**, onc-t., paeon., phyt., **Puls.**, **Sabad.**, sul-ac., *thuj.*

Back

- STIFFNESS; Muscles; erector spinae, when rising from bed, when coughing (1): aq-get.

Compare Related Remedies

- Asafoetida, Angostura vera, Fluoric acid and Nitric acid, Lithium carbonicum, Strontium carbonicum, Silicea terra.

Related Levels

- Syphilitic Miasm.
- Clinical Rubric Clusters.

Generalities

- ULCERS; bones, periosteum; discharge, with putrid (5): **Aq-Get.**, **Asaf.**, *merc.*, *ph-ac.*, **Sil.**
- CARIES, necrosis; bones; long (18): **ANG.**, **Aq-Get.**, **Asaf.**, **Aur.**, ba-sv., **Calc.**, dros., **Fl-ac.**, hecla., kali-bi., **Lith-c.**, mez., morg., **Nit-ac.**, *sec.*, **SIL.**, **Still.**, **Stront-c.**

Extremities

- CARIES, necrosis; Hips (10): **Ang.**, **Aq-Get.**, **Asaf.**, **Aur.**, **Fl-ac.**, hecla., **Lith-c.**, **Nit-ac.**, **Sil.**, **STRONT-C.**
- CARIES, necrosis; Thighs; bones, femur (10): **Ang.**, **Aq-Get.**, **Asaf.**, **Aur.**, **Fl-ac.**, hecla., **Lith-c.**, **Nit-ac.**, **Sil.**, **STRONT-C.**

CASE 6.1 Polymyalgia Rheumatica

Context

An overweight woman of 50 with mousy brown curly hair who sits very still with her hands held together.

Consultation August 1999

I feel so tired all the time I've been diagnosed with depression and am on Prozac. And I have heavy painful periods. I was prescribed hormone treatment for the period pain and since then I've been depressed and ended up on Prozac. My periods are only occasional now.

I'm so anxious about my health – I just can't cope. I get shaky. I can't bear people to see that I get shaky. I work in a bank so people can see my hands and they look at them when they shake. I work as a cashier. I seem to get silly spells where I make mistakes and the cash doesn't balance. Sometimes I just can't seem to concentrate. My self confidence has gone way down I'm so self conscious. I shake inside here. . . .

(Observation: Puts hand on epigastrium.) . . . as well as my hands.

I get hot flushes sweats all day long – worse when it's hot and humid. I get about 12 flushes a day. I wake at night at about 3.30 or 4 a.m. It's worse when my periods are due even though the period may not arrive. The flush starts here (*Observation: puts hand on epigastrium*) and goes upwards over my head and then comes the sweat.

I keep getting virus infections with big glands in my neck and earache and headaches and a tickly cough. It seems to recur with 2 weeks off in between. My energy is 50/100 – I'm dreadful in the morning – just exhausted I can't concentrate. Then the energy creeps up by lunch time and then I have slump between 4–6 p.m., then I'm ready for bed by 10pm.

I had measles very badly when I was 6 – I was off school for 5 weeks. Then I went back to school for 3 days, got severe food poisoning and nearly died. I came out in big blebs all over my skin – I still remember the itch it was so awful. I was off school for 6 weeks. After that I got lots of colic. I had bad glandular fever and got jaundice with it. I had my appendix taken out when I was 16. I had pertussis when I was 9, mumps when I was 12 but they were OK. I had severe chicken pox at 31. As a teenager I had lots of tonsillitis and had my tonsils out at 17.

I've had 3 children and a miscarriage. I've had an ovarian cyst and an ovary removed. I fractured my nose in a car crash and got lots of sinusitis after that and then had an operation on my nose, and then I was OK.

I'm a farmer's wife. My parents were strict, teetotallers and church-goers. My childhood, teens and young life as a woman were via the church and its social life. I met my husband there. My father died of gangrene of his feet aged 87 and my mother of multiple strokes at 83. I've 2 older brothers.

I always have very cold feet all year round – they are as cold as stone – I can't sleep if my feet are too cold. I'm worse from the heat of the sun – I can't stand it – I can't work in the garden if it's hot sunny – it saps my energy I feel sick. I have to wear a hat and sunglasses. I usually just sit in the shade. I get a headache before thunderstorms. My stomach gets upset if it's very cold frosty. I get heartburn from dried fruit, cucumber, pastry and onions. I love sweets and rice puddings.

Observation: *She sits still, makes few gestures – she is overweight.* I seem to spend my life hurrying yet I diddle about till the last minute then have to rush then I end up being late. I am very worried about my health. I worry about money. There is a little niggling background worry that we will have to sell the farm and have nowhere to go.

I had depression in the past – 13 years ago. It lasted for years. Yes I've been depressed on and off since with a few years gap. I was on Prozac for 4 years after my father died. I'm terrified of rats and mice – just like my mother. I am sacred of heights and feel wobbly looking out from a height – I would have to stay away from the edge.

Analysis: symptom pattern clear the symptoms fit 1 pattern with no apparent obstacle to healing.

Management

Calcarea carbonica 30c day 1, 200c day 2, 1M day 3, then 12c daily.

Consultation September 1999 (6 weeks later)

I do feel a bit better – I've more drive more motivation my energy is clearly better – it's 70/100 now. I still have plenty of hot sweats, but my sleep is OK – I'm waking up less often, lately only occasionally. I wake up feeling better – I don't wake feeling dreadful or feeling sickly. I still get the slump in energy from 4–6 and still go to bed at 10. There is less anxiety depression shakiness – I've definitely been less shaky.

Observation: Scores amelioration as 75% on visual analogue scale.

Management

Continue Calcarea carbonica 12c daily till off Prozac then take it as required for acute illnesses and return when needs to.

Consultation November 2013

I was diagnosed with fibromyalgia 3 years ago and more recently the diagnosis has changed to polymyalgia rheumatica. I had shingles 2 months ago and have been awful since. I always seem to be ill keep getting virus illnesses then this shingles has been the last straw. The blisters came out on the left side of my neck and the top of my shoulder. My GP prescribed acyclovir – the rash went away in 3 days, but I have felt awful ill since then. The pain is back in my left neck and shoulder. Each time I get the virus thing I get such sore muscles or sore bits of muscles. They are sore, sore to touch and ache all the time. I feel so awful I just have to go to bed to rest – that is the only thing that will help.

My energy is 10/100 on bad days when I wake in the mornings then crawls up to 30/100. From 10 till about 3 I can potter about and get things done and then my energy slumps back down to 10/100 again. I've been prescribed pregabalin and have taken it for 2 years; sertraline because of my anxiety and lansoprazole for the burning in my gullet, and I take paracetamol regularly for the muscle pain.

Analysis

Change in illness = new remedy required.

Recurrent "viral" illnesses and echoes herald a new auto-immune disease – needs a bowel nosode to restore bowel flora and raise immunity – Bacillus no. 7 (Paterson) has the most fatigue.

Then Calcarea carbonica again as it helped so much before. She continues to sit still all the time – never fidgets, never moves – she sits like she was poured.

Management

Bacillus no. 7 30c daily for 3 days wait 2 weeks, then Calcarea carbonica 1M 1 dose then LM1 2 drops daily in water.

Outcome to January 2014
No change – treatment: Carcinosin 30c 1 dose daily for 3 days then wait 3 weeks then Morgan Pure 30c 1 dose daily for 3 days then wait 3 weeks then Herpes zoster nosode 30c 1 dose daily for 3 days with Calcarea carbonica LM1 daily on all the days not taking a nosode. Consider sending bloods for food intolerance tests (IgM antibodies – York labs).

Consultation 7 April 2014
I felt better for a few days with each of the new medicines a bit better the last few days but overall there has been little change. BUT I was very ill in March with pleurisy ended up on two courses of antibiotics. I woke up in the early morning 1 day in March with shaking chills such a sore back chest on the left side felt so hot so very ill. My GP sent me to hospital. I was there for a few days and then discharged on antibiotics and had 2 whole courses. I am exhausted since then and all my muscles are so sore all the time.

On examination: chest clear, no pleural rub. Muscles of neck and shoulders feel stiff and hard and are a little tender. The inter-costal muscles of her right lower chest feel stiff and hard.

Analysis

- Polymyalgia rheumatic is a new illness with a new symptom pattern needs a new remedy.
- She is still immune suppressed, needs a bowel nosode especially after all the antibiotics.
- Remedy pattern recognised.

Management

Morgan Pure 30c 1 dose daily 3 days then Aqua Gettysburg LM1, 2 drops daily in water with 10 succusions before each dose.

Rubrics – retrospective, using Complete Repertory 2015 of Van Zanvoort.[1]

Generalities

- Stiffness, rigidity; muscles (73).**
- Lying; ameliorates; during; quietly (36).*

Extremities

- Stiffness; lying quietly ameliorates (1): aq-get.
- Pain; rheumatic; rest; ameliorates (2): aq-get., bry.

Generalities

- Exercise, exertion; aversion to (44).
- Pain; rheumatic; motion; aggravates (59).*

Back

- Stiffness; cervical region (353).

Mind

- Work; mental; aversion to (312).
- Indolence, aversion to work (548).

Chest

- Pain; sides; left; inspiration; aggravates (40).

The reperotisation matrix generated by MacRepertory is shown in Figure 6.1.

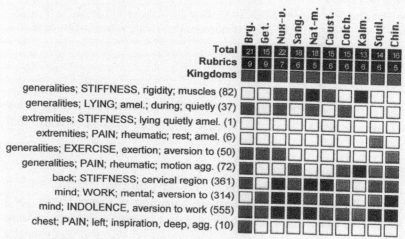

Figure 6.1 Matrix generated by MacRepertory using Complete Repertory 2015 Van Zandvoort.[1]

Consultation June 2014

My bowels went a bit loose with some griping pain and diarrhoea 3 times, then it was over and then my fibromyalgia flared up a bit, but overall I have been better.

Observation: Now she is calling her illness fibromyalgia again not polymyalgia rheumatica.

There are just not so many days when I'm feeling bad. I'm doing more. I get better as the day goes on and by evening I'm still doing things about the house. I'm not picking up every virus illness that's going around. I have less spells in bed with bad fibromyalgia pains. I was in bed yesterday for the 1st time since I was here but I'm not so bad today – usually the flare ups last longer. There has been a little but clear shift.

The York labs tests were strongly positive for cow's milk and yeast, so I've been having Greek Feta and soya yoghurts and I enjoy them.

Management

The patient was asked to continue Aqua Gettysburg LM1, 2 drops daily and all usual drugs.

Consultation September 2014

Overall, I've been quite good. I'm still not picking up all the viral illnesses going around. The fibromyalgia continues and gets bad for a day and I go to bed, but that used to last 3 days to a week. I get bursts of energy then get tired need to rest. If I overdo it the next day I'm useless and need to rest.

Management

The patient was encouraged to try walking for 30 minutes each day – continue Aqua Gettysburg LM1, 2 drops daily and all conventional drugs.

Consultation April 2015

On Christmas day I came down with flu – proper influenza – I was exhausted aching headache, hot and sweating and went to bed for a week. I was ill for 3–4 weeks. In January I had an operation because I was leaking from my breast – they removed the milk duct with a benign polyp in it. I'm still off cow's milk and yeast but I just feel stuck since the flu. I really struggle in the mornings. I wake at 6 to pee then go straight back to sleep. When I waken later it's a real struggle again. I feel cold all the time all over my body but especially my back and am still waking soaked with sweat during the night.

Analysis

Slow convalescence and incomplete recovery after influenza – needs an inter-current remedy and rise in potency of Aqua Gettysburg.

Management

Carcinosin 30C 1 dose daily for 3 days then Aqua Gettysburg LM2 as 2 drops daily. If better to try reducing pregabalin from 1 morning 2 at night to 1 twice a day.

Consultation July 2015

I was better for a while, but I'm exhausted all the time again. The fibromyalgia is rotten. I've had a head cold, bunged sinuses, catarrh and a bad stabbing pain in my left ear – it comes suddenly stabs straight in.

Observation: This pain is typical of jaw joint dysfunction.

On examination: left tympanic membrane normal. There is full range of movement of left jaw joint but very tender and rigid, hard muscles around left jaw joint.

Advice

Remedial massage.

My energy has gone down to 50/100. After gardening for an hour I ache all over the next day. I feel worse in hot, humid weather and in very cold weather. I feel cold all the time all down my back and all through my body again and still get some sweats. Yes, I'm taking pregabalin 1 tablet twice a day.

Management

Carcinosin 30C, one dose daily for 3 days once a month for 3 months with Aqua Gettysburg LM2, 2 drops daily 27 days/month.

Consultation October 2015

I'm not so bad at all really. I had another cold 4 weeks ago but didn't need to go to bed. I've only needed 1 day in bed 2 weeks ago. This morning I had the cold feeling through my body again. My bowels have been a bit loose and watery for a while – I've not had a diarrhoea illness or a viral thing but my bowels are just a bit loose watery most days. My energy is 75/100 most days. 1 hour gardening is still long enough – any longer my muscles ache in my back and pelvis and hips. I've looked after my grandchildren lots during the summer holidays – three boys aged 10, 9, and 7. I've enjoyed it and been OK. I've stayed of yeast and cow's milk for 18 months must I continue to stay off them? If I have custard with cow's milk or a sandwich I feel worse, my tummy feels bad.

Analysis

Significant improvement in polymyalgia rheumatic continues but current bowel symptoms which persist.

Management

Polybowel nosode 30c, one dose daily for 3 days and then continue Aqua Gettysburg LM2, 2 drops daily.

AQUA HALL

Source

The salt springs of Hall in Austria.

Contents

The springs contain chlorides, iodides, bromides, carbonates of the alkaline earth metals plus iron as ferrous salts – the main constituent is sodium chloride.

Compare with: Nat-muriaticum, but *Aqua Hall* has no issues about sun, sea or salt.

Rubrics

Sensitivity and vulnerability: emotional and cognitive – loss of resilience – overwhelm

- Chest; FALLING; off, as if, mammae (1): aq-hall.
- Stomach; FALL out, as if would (6): aq-hall, bell., cact., lyc., *mag-c.*, ox-ac.
- Neck; TENSION; Thyroid gland (4): agar., aq-hall, calc-f, *iod.*, lat-m.

Suppression of emotions – Sublimation of libido

Chest

- PAIN; itching; nipples; rubbing ameliorates (1): aq-hall.
- PAIN; burning, smarting; mammae; nipples; left; itching, rubbing ameliorates (1): aq-hall.

- Abdomen; PAIN; circular, around umbilicus (1): aq-hall.
- Extremities; PAIN; stitching; needles, as from; feet; heels; right (1): aq-hall.
- Respiration; DIFFICULT; menses; before (19).

Clinical Rubric Clusters

Breasts – sensitive, painful, heavy, as if will fall off

- Especially left breast left nipple – very sensitive.

- Pain: burning stitching itching, worse from touch and motion, ameliorated by rubbing.
- Sensation of heaviness.
- Atrophy, falling of breasts in young women.

Chest; PAIN; Ulcerative

- Mammae: night (1): aq-hall.
- Mammae: motion aggravates (1): aq-hall.
- Mammae: touch aggravates (1): aq-hall.
- PAIN: Itching; nipples; rubbing ameliorates (1): aq-hall.

- SENSITIVE; mammae: night (1): aq-hall motion aggravates (1): aq-hall.
- HEAVINESS: Mammae; motion touch aggravates (1): aq-hall.

Headaches

PAIN, headache

- Transient; occiput (1): aq-hall.
- Drawing; vertex; extending to; temple; right (1): aq-hall.
- Tearing; vertex; extending; temples, over; right (1): aq-hall.
- Tearing; vertex; extending; temples, over (2): ang., aq-hall.
- Drawing; vertex; extending to; temple (3): aq-hall, bor., chel.
- Vertex; extending to; temples (15): *amet.*, ang., aq-hall, arg., bor., bry., carb-v., caust., cham., chel., hell., hipp., kalm., phos., uran.

Swelling lymph nodes

Neck

- SWELLING; painless, lymphatic tissue (5): aq-hall, Calc., hippoz., Ign., med.

Chest

- SENSITIVE; lymphatic tissue, axillae (5): aq-hall, lob-e., nit-ac., rhus-r., sul-ac.

Generalities

- SWELLING; painless; glands, liver, spleen (25).

Respiratory Tract Infection

Nose

- INFLAMMATION; catarrhal; evening; cough, during dry (1): aq-hall.
- INFLAMMATION; catarrhal; evening (7): adam., ant-t., aq-hall, **Carb-an.**, hydrog., mang., **Puls.**

Throat

- MUCOUS, discharges; hoarseness, with (4): aq-hall, *arg-n.*, lach., *nat-m.*

Speech and voice

- HOARSENESS; scraping in throat, with (9): alum., **Anag.**, aq-hall, **CAUST.**, cimic., **Kreos.**, **Mez.**, **Nux-v.**, puls.

Irritable bowel syndrome

Stomach

- PAIN; corrosive, gnawing; extending to; downward (1): aq-hall.

Abdomen

- RUMBLING noise; stool, as before (3): ant-t., aq-hall, m-art.
- PAIN; cramping, gripping; umbilical region.
- Right (2): aq-hall, merc-c.
- PAIN; cutting; umbilical region; extending to: rectum (2): aloe, aq-hall.
- PAIN; cutting; umbilical region; extending downward (3): aq-hall, **Coloc.**, ip.

Skin – Boils – burning upon touch

Skin

- ERUPTIONS; boils, furuncles; burning; touch, on (1): aq-hall.

Chest

- ERUPTIONS; boils, furuncles; mammae (5): am-c., aq-hall, chin., mag-c., phos.

Extremities

- ERUPTIONS; boils, furuncles; upper arms; right (1): aq-hall.
- ERUPTIONS; boils, furuncles; elbow, right (2): aq-hall, lach.
- PAIN; burning, smarting; forearms; skin, external (4): aq-hall, aur-m-n., con., mur-ac.
- ERUPTIONS; night (13): aq-hall, arg-n., arum-t., *bacch-a.*, **Merc.**, oxpr., phos., pitu-a., **Pix.**, **Psor.**, puls-n., strep-s., term-a.

Other Unique Rubrics of Aqua Hall

Chest

- PAIN; axilla; right; stretching out arm (1): aq-hall.

Extremities

- PAIN; drawing; upper arms; bones, humerus: left.
- PAIN; drawing; upper arms; bones, humerus; extending to, elbow.

Related Remedies
Aqua Marina, Senecio aureus, Silica ferra, Iodine, Thyroidinum.

Level = Clinical Rubric Clusters

Aqua Marina

Chest

- PAIN; sternum; night; aggravates (14): am-c., aq-hall, aq-mar., aur., **Chel.**, chin., cinch., ferr., hydrc., merc-c., ozone, petr., stram., stront-c.

Senecio aureus, Silicea terra

Chest

- PAIN; burning, smarting; mammae; nipples; left (6): aq-hall, sac-l., **Senec.**, **SIL.**, spira., zinc.
- PAIN; burning, smarting; mammae; left (14): ambr., ant-t., aq-hall. chin-ar., herin., indg., lyc., phos., sac-l., **Senec.**, **SIL.**, spira., tax-br., zinc.

Iodine, Thyroidinum

Neck

- TENSION; Thyroid gland (4): agar., aq-hall, calc-f, *iod.*, lat-m.

Chest

- FLABBY mammae (15): **Acon.**, aq-hall, bell., calc., cham., **CON.**, hydr., **IOD.**, kali-i., kreos., nit-ac., nux-m., onos., **Thyr.**, verat-v.

AQUA HOCHSTEIN

Source

An ambient mineral spring rising in the national park at Passau in Ilztal in Germany.

Proving

Proving done in 1996 by Hans Eberle and Friedrich Ritzer.[2]

Rubrics

Sensitivity and vulnerability: emotional and cognitive – loss of resilience – overwhelm

Sensitive and vulnerable yet functioning

- QUICK to act; waking, on (3): *aq-hoch., lac-h.*, lac-mat.
- MUSIC; desires; compose, to (2): aq-hoch., pras-o.
- INTUITIVE (14): acon., *amet.*, aq-hoch., aquilr-a., bar-c., cann-i., ilx-p., lac-leo., plut-n., pras-c., pras-o., sep., spect., terb.

- Thoughts: clarity – abundance – mischievous.
- Relaxed feeling, letting go.
- Mildness, quiet disposition.
- Affectionate yet impressionable and susceptible.

- COMMUNICATIVE, expansive; alternating with taciturn (1): aq-hoch.
- MILDNESS; alternating with; hardness (3): *aq-hoch.*, croc., scorp.

Dreams

- Overlooked, being (1): *aq-hoch.*
- Needed, he is not (1): aq-hoch.
- Rooms, of; empty (2): aq-hoch., cordy-a.
- Relationships; bad (1): aq-hoch.
- Relationships (4): aq-hoch., lap-be-e., *ros-ca.*, soph-m.

Ailments from (smaller rubrics examples)

- FRIGHT, fear; accident, from sight of an (4): **ACON.**, *aq-hoch.*, **Calc.**, carb-v., **OP.**
- GRIEF; financial loss, from (8): *aq-hoch.*, **Arn.**, ars., **Aur.**, mangi., **Mez.**, pras-o., **Psor.**
- DISCORDS, relatives, friends, between; parents (12): acon., **Ant-t.**, *aq-hoch.*, bufo, chr., gado-n., gado-p., holm., lant-c., plac., *plut-n.*, prot.

Ailments from

- Love; disappointment/or unhappy.
- Disappointment, deception.
- Death; loved ones, of – parents or friends, of.
- Embarrassment, humiliation, mortification.
- Injuries accidents, violence, vehemence.
- Abuse/domination by others.

- DEPENDENT; sexual, erotic (2): aq-hoch., electr. (So needy so vulnerable to allow the above to happen to continue.)
- SADNESS: separation from friends, family aggravates (6): *aq-hoch.*, cer-p., excr-can., holm-c., *nic-r.*, plac.

Loss of Resilience, emotional and cognitive

- REPROACHES; oneself; neglecting her children (1): aq-hoch.
- IRRITABILITY; women, towards (1): aq-hoch.
- PERSONS, aversion to; certain; smokers (1): aq-hoch.
- RESERVED; partner, towards (2): aq-hoch., haliae-lc.

- ANXIETY; abortion; after (5): aq-hoch., **Cimic.**, excr-can., **Op.**, **Sabin.**
- ABORTION; ailments from, aggravates (9): aq-hoch., **Caul.**, **Cimic.**, excr-can., helon., lac-ory., **Op.**, ruta, **Sabin.**

Skin

- GOOSE flesh; Fear, fright, from (2): aq-hoch., **GELS.**
- GOOSE flesh; Sudden, hair standing on end, during chill (5): aq-hoch., bar-c., dulc., meny., uran-n.

- FEAR; dentist, of going to (6): *aq-hoch.*, calc., lyc., nat-glut., puls., tub.
- IRRESOLUTION, indecision; life choices, about big (8): *aq-hoch.*, cer-s., des-ac., gado-n., kali-sil., lac-dr., pras., pter-a.
- IRRESOLUTION, indecision; marry, to (14): *aq-hoch.*, carb-v., ign., lach., lyc., nat-m., nux-v., phos., plat., pras-c., sil., sile-c., staph., verat.

- QUARRELSOMENESS, scolding; family, with his; husband, to (7): *amet.*, *aq-hoch.*, calop-s., haliae-lc., hyos., lac-lup., **Thuj.**
- ANGER; family, toward; mother, mother-in-law (9): *aq-hoch.*, cer-c., excr-can., lac-dr., lant-c., lant-o., scorp., thul-f., thul-m.
- HATRED; mother, of (10): aq-hoch., *excr-can.*, hell., nat-m., peg-h., plac., raph., sama-m., *scorp.*, thul-o.
- MEDDLESOME (11): alco., alum., aq-hoch., atro., aur-s., **Chel.**, con., *hyos.*, hyosin., lyc., plb.

Overwhelm

Sleep

- SLEEPLESSNESS; divorce, after (1): aq-hoch.
- RISE; must; sleeplessness, from (5): aq-hoch., con., **Nux-v.**, phos., **Rhus-t.**
- SLEEPLESSNESS; wide awake (10): aq-hoch., aur., calc., cham., chin., coff., gels., kali-i., sulph., valer.

- SLEEPLESSNESS; grief, after (14): *aq-hoch.*, aur., carc., **COLOC.**, **Gels.**, graph., **Ign.**, **Kali-br.**, lach., **NAT-M.**, op., **Sulph.**, uran., zinc-val.

- DELUSIONS, imaginations: Partner, will not find a new (1): aq-hoch.
- ESTRANGED; husband, from her (5): aids, aq-hoch., culx-p., hydr-ac., *thuj.*
- SUICIDAL disposition; love disappointment, from (8): ant-c., aq-hoch., **Aur.**, **Bell.**, **Caust.**, **Hyos.**, plut-n., **Staph.**
- MARRIAGE; aversion to; idea of marriage seemed unendurable (10): *aq-hoch.*, gado-m., **Lach.**, lyc., **Med.**, nux-v., pic-ac., puls., staph., tub.

Suppression of emotions – Sublimation of libido

- QUARRELSOMENESS, scolding; waking, on (6): aq-hoch., carc., cupr-acet., **Lyc.**, nux-v., petr.
- Vertigo; DIVORCE, from (1): aq-hoch.
- Female; Sexual libido; desire diminished; wanting; nursing mothers, in (1): aq-hoch.

- CONFUSION of mind; love, disappointed, aggravates (1): aq-hoch.
- CONFUSION of mind; emotions, about (4): *aq-hoch.*, clem., polyst., pter-a.

- DETACHED; relationships, from emotional (5): aq-hoch., erb., iod., lute., stan-e.
- DETACHED; family, home, from (8): aq-hoch., coriand., erb., heli., iod., lute., *pot-a.*, stan-e.

Exhaustion – mental and physical

- DREAMS; money; problems, with (3): aq-hoch., hema-h., lac-eq.
- FINANCE; inaptitude for (6): aq-hoch., ars., cypra-e., lyc., puls., **SIL.**
- NEGLECTS; everything (6): am-c., *aq-hoch.*, bar-c., caust., tell., ytte.
- BUSINESS; neglects his (9): *aq-hoch.*, *cassi-s.*, lac-lup., lim-b-c., opun-v., ptel., salx-f., **Sulph.**, ytte.

- TELEVISION watching; aggravates, ailments from (1): aq-hoch.
- TELEVISION watching; desires (3): *adon.*, aq-hoch., lac-as.
- COMPUTERS, electronic games; desires (6): *aq-hoch.*, calc-i., euro-n., excr-can., thul., ytte-p.

Children

- DREAMS; parents, of; parents divorce (3): aq-hoch., germ., naja-m.
- DIVORCE, ailments from, aggravates; children, in (10): aeth., *aq-hoch.*, cer-c., cycl., dysp-n., excr-can., holm-o., lant-c., lant-o., nat-m.

- KICKS; child is cross, kicks and scolds, waking, on (2): aq-hoch., **Lyc.,**
- ABSENT-MINDEDNESS; children, in (2): *aq-hoch.*, bac.
- WEANING, ailments from (2): aq-hoch., lac-h.

Bladder

- RETENTION of urine; colic, in (5): aq-hoch., arn., **Coloc.**, **PLB.**, thuj.

- Dreams; water; waterworks (1): aq-hoch.
- Dreams; animals, of; swept away by water (1): aq-hoch.
- Stomach; thirst; night, waking, on (19).**

Clinical Rubric Clusters

'Never well since' – Glandular fever

Generalities

- MONONUCLEOSIS, after effects of (11): ail., aq-mar., aq-hoch., bar-c., bar-m., calen., carc., crot-c., foll., gali., *thuj.*

Sliding into hypomania?
- HEEDLESS, careless; money matters, in (1): aq-hoch.
- RICH; fancies himself (1): aq-hoch.
- DELUSIONS, imaginations; cheap, things are (1): aq-hoch.
- CHAOTIC; life (4): *aq-hoch.*, neod-c., *plut-n.*, pras-m.
- KLEPTOMANIA; steals; money (3): *aq-hoch.*, calc., puls.

If the patient has the first four symptoms then the possibility of a diagnosis of Bi-Polar Disorder must be considered and an appropriate referral made.

Vertigo Divorce, from (1): aq-hoch

Tonsillitis and Diphtheria (in diphtheria as supportive treatment or for never well since)

Throat

- BLACK (7): aq-hoch., bism., carb-v., **Echi.**, merc-c., merc-d., merc-s.
- GREY (8): aq-hoch., aq-sanic., **Iod.**, **Kali-m.**, lyc., **Merc-cy.**, phel., **Phyt.**
- DEPOSITS, tonsils; greyish (12): ail., apis, aq-hoch., echi., kali-m., lac-c., merc., merc-c., **Merc-i-r.**, **Mur-ac.**, phyt., sabad.

Heartburn

Stomach

- HEARTBURN; bananas, after (1): aq-hoch.
- HEARTBURN; tea; ameliorates (1): aq-hoch.

Heart, circulation

- PAIN: heart region; eating, after (13): aq-hoch., aspar., chin-s., erech., **Kali-bi.**, **Lil-t.**, lyc., mag-c., magn-gr., manc., *meny.*, nat-m., stront-c.

Useful and/or Unusual Rubrics

Generalities

- TINGLING, prickling; heated, on becoming (2): aq-hoch., atp.
- SWIMMING; desires (7): *aq-hoch.*, bute-j., cyg-c., geoc-c., hema-h., lac-del., onc-t.

Nose

- EPISTAXIS, haemorrhage; vomiting; with (5): aq-hoch., *ars.*, dros., **Ox-ac.**, sars.

Chest

- INFLAMMATION; recurrent; lungs (6): aq-hoch., bac., **Erio.**, **Ferr-p.**, **Kali-n.**, med.
- PAIN; flatus; ameliorates (6): aq-hoch., meny., mur-ac., ph-ac., sol, stram.

Back

- NUMBNESS, insensibility; sacral region (9): *acon.*, aq-hoch., *berb.*, **Calc-p.**, *carb-v.*, **Graph.**, ox-ac., plat., *spong.*
- NUMBNESS, insensibility; sacral region; lower limbs, and (3): aq-hoch., **Calc-p.**, **Graph.**

Extremities

CRACKS, fissures; bleeding:

- Fingers; tips (3): aq-hoch., rhus-v., ulm-c.
- Fingers (5): aq-hoch., ars., lac-v-b., rhus-v., ulm-c.

Compare Related remedies

Aqua Sanicula, Aqua Taosca, Ignatia amara, Aqua Hochstein and Gemstone and Rose, Aqua Hochstein and Gemstone and Milk and Energy and Actinide and Lanthanide.

Aqua Sanicula, Aqua Taosca

- KICKS: child is cross, kicks and scolds (11): aq-hoch., **Aq-Sanic.**, bufo, **CHAM.**, cina, cupr., kreos., **Lyc.**, *plut-n.*, psor., scorp.

Ears

- PAIN; bathing, washing; aggravates (3): *aq-hoch.*, aq-taosc., cortico.

Ignatia amara

Sleep

- RESTLESS; mortification, from (2): aq-hoch., **Ign.**
- SLEEPLESSNESS; grief, after (14): *aq-hoch.*, aur., carc., **COLOC.**, **Gels.**, graph., **Ign.**, **Kali-br.**, lach., **NAT-M.**, op., **Sulph.**, uran., zinc-val.

Aqua Hochstein and Gemstone and Rose

- DREAMS; Relationships (4): aq-hoch., lap-be-e., *ros-ca.*, soph-m.

Aqua Hochstein and Gemstone and Milk and Energy and Actinide and Lanthanides

- INTUITIVE (14): acon., *amet.*, aq-hoch., aquilr-a., bar-c., cann-i., ilx-p., lac-leo., plut-n., pras-c., pras-o., sep., spect., terb.

Aqua Hochstein and Gemstone and Bird and Milk

- QUARRELSOMENESS, scolding; family, with his; husband, to (7): *amet.*, *aq-hoch.*, calop-s., haliae-lc., hyos., lac-lup., **Thuj.**

AQUA JATZFELD

Source

A spring rising at Jatzfeld Soolbad in Wurtemburg, Germany.

Contents

The analysis of contents of the spring has been lost. The town still exists but is not a spa.

Rubrics

Clinical Rubric Clusters

Inflammation and hard swelling of lymph nodes, spleen and exocrine glands

Mouth

- HARDNESS; glands, salivary; submaxillary, submandibulary (36): . . . *aq-jatz.*, . . . **BAR-C.**, **BAR-M.**, **Brom.**, **Carb-v.**, clem., **Cocc.**, **Con.**, **Cupr.**,

... **Iod**. . . **Merc-i-f** . . . **Phyt**. . . **Psor.**, **Rhus-t.**, sarr., sil., spig., **Spong**. . . **Syph.**, trif-r., tub.

Generalities

- **SWELLING******: Glands, liver, spleen. . . ******; Lymphatic tissue******; Oedematous******; Hard****** Hard, glands, liver, spleen.******

Face

- GLANDS, salivary******; Submaxillary, submandibular.******

Mouth

- INDURATION SWELLING: Glands, salivary******; submandibular.******

Neck

- INDURATION,****** SWELLING: Lymphatic tissue, cervical.******

Ulcers

Extremities

- ULCERS; feet; heels (19): **All-c.**, am-c., **Am-m.**, anac., *aq-jatz.*, aran., **Ars.**, arund., bor., **CAUST.**, echi., kali-bi., lach., lam., laur., **NAT-C.**, **Paeon.**, **SEP.**, **SIL.**

Tuberculosis (as supportive treatment)

Skin

- ERUPTIONS; tuberculous (21): **Aethi-a.**, aln., *aq-jatz.*, bac., bar-c., **Bov.**, brom., **Calc.**, calc-p., con., cory., **Iod.**, merc., mez., **Sarr.**, sil., **Sol-n.**, **Solid.**, **Sulph.**, tub., viol-t.

Generalities

- SWELLING; tuberculous (47): . . . aq-elmen, aq-get., *aq-jatz.*, **Ars.**, **Brom.**, **CALC.**, **Calc-i.**, **Cist.**, . . . **Ferr.**, **IOD.**, **Lyc.**, **PULS.**, . . . **Scroph-n.**, **Sil.**, **Stann.**, **Stront-c.**, **SULPH.**

AQUA KISSINGEN

Source

The Rakoczy Spring of Kissingen Spa in Bavaria is a cold, salty and gaseous spring.

Contents

The spring contains mainly sodium chloride with traces of other chloride salts plus dissolved nitrogen and oxygen gases.

The remedy is made from the water – symptoms from drinking the water and bathing in the spa.

Compare with: Natrum muriaticum – Aqua Kissingen has no issues about sun or sea or salt.

Compare with: Calcarea carbonica – Horrible sights stories profoundly affect; anxiety in pit of stomach; cannot bear to be looked at.

Rubrics

Sensitivity and vulnerability: emotional and cognitive – loss of resilience – overwhelm

* STARTING, startled; Electric shock, as from; sleep; falling asleep, on (1): aq-kiss.
* STARTING, startled; electric shock, as from (12): agar., aq-kiss., **Arg.**, **Ars.**, cann-s., euph., lsd, mag-m., **Nat-m.**, nat-p., *nux-m.*, stram.

* WEARY of life; sudden (1): aq-kiss.
* ANGUISH; night; waking, on (4): aq-kiss., kali-br., **Nat-s.**, **Nux-v.**
* THOUGHTS; persistent; frightful; night; waking, on (3): aq-kiss., phys., **Visc.**
* THOUGHTS; persistent; frightful; night (7): aq-kiss., hydr., kali-br., op., phos., phys., **Visc.**
* RESTLESSNESS, nervousness; night; waking (7): agar., aq-kiss., caust., lyc., par., saroth., sep.
* FRIGHTENED easily; night; waking, on (13): aq-kiss., **ARS.**, bufo, cham., *cina*, con., **Euphr.**, lat-h., m-arct., m-aust., **Psor.**, **Sep.**, **Sol-t-ae.**

Sleep

* WAKING; frequent; restlessness, with (8): aq-kiss., aran., haliae-lc., **Lach.**, latex, m-aust., nicc., **Puls.**

* WEEPING, tearful mood; looking at anyone (1): aq-kiss.
* WEEPING, tearful mood; looked at, when (8): **Ant-c.**, ant-t., aq-kiss., brom., cina, **Nat-m.**, staph., **Tarent.**
* WEEPING, tearful mood; lamenting, moaning, and (7): acon., aq-kiss., brom., **Coff.**, *hell.*, op., sabad.

* DESIRES: unpleasant things, to think about (1): aq-kiss.

- BROODING; cares, worries, unpleasant things (6): aq-kiss., **Aur.**, **Ign.**, nitro., ros-g., staph.
- DWELLS; Events, on past disagreeable.

Suppression of emotions – Sublimation of libido

- Nose; FORMICATION, crawling; right (2): aq-kiss., **Teucr.**
- Kidneys; FORMICATION, crawling (5): aq-kiss., brach., dirc., hydrc., med.
- Abdomen; RETRACTION; Convulsive, spasmodic (9): *act-sp.*, aq-kiss., *chel.*, *plat.*, plb., plb-chr., stram., **Sul-ac.**, *tab.*
- Abdomen; CONSTRICTION; inguinal region (10): aq-kiss., bov., **Cact.**, **Cimic.**, eug., gamb., kali-n., macrin., mag-c., rat.

Clinical Rubric Clusters

Sadness and depression in yielding children who after a fright:

- Become anxious, startle as from shock when falling asleep.
- Cannot bear to be looked at.
- Withdraw into a morose silent brooding state.
- Sink into depression with twitching eyelids especially right lower lid.

Face pain – Trigeminal Neuralgia

Face

- PAIN; pressing; asunder; cheek bones (4): aq-kiss., colch., merc., **Thuj.**
- PAIN; burning, smarting; lips; upper; night (1): aq-kiss.
- SWELLING; lips; upper; night (1): aq-kiss.

Useful or Unusual Rubrics

Stool

- ASAFOETIDA, smell like (2): aq-kiss., cic.

Compare/Related Remedies

Aqua Sanicula, Aqua Kissingen and Energy Remedies, Aqua Kissingen and Gemstones, Aqua Kissingen and Lanthanides.
Clinical Rubric Cluster level.

Aqua Sanicula

Chill

- POSTPONING, belated (12): alst-s., aq-kiss., aq-sanic., bry., *canth.*, chin., cina, **GAMB.**, ign., **Ip.**, kali-bi., phos.

Aqua Kissingen and Energy Remedies

Extremities

- INFLAMMATION; hands; back (3): aq-kiss., kali-m., m-arct.

Head

- CONGESTION, hyperaemia; Coldness of extremities, with: Feet (3): aq-kiss., m-arct., phyt.

Mouth

- PAIN; stitching; tongue; edges (9): *ant-c.*, apis, aq-kiss., brass., *m-aust.*, mang-acet., nux-v., ph-ac., *staph.*

Aqua Kissingen and Gemstones

Mouth

- TINGLING, prickling; tongue; edges, margins (4): aq-kiss., lach., lap-be-e., ped.

Aqua Kissingen and Lanthanides

Vision

- DIPLOPIA; headache; with (8): aq-kiss., **Gels.**, ger., kali-chl., morph-m., neod-s., phyt., stroph.

AQUA KRONTHAL

Source

A spring rising in the spa town of Bad Kronthal near Frankfurt, Germany.

Content[3]

- Row 2: Lithium salt traces, carbonic acid.
- Row 3: Sodium chloride, sodium carbonate, magnesium carbonate, silica.
- Row 4: Potassium chloride, potassium sulphate, calcium carbonate, ferrous carbonate, manganese salt traces.
- Row 5: Strontium salt traces.
- Row 6: Barium salt traces.

Compare: Agnus castus at level of Clinical Rubric Clusters.

Rubrics

Sensitivity and vulnerability: emotional and cognitive – loss of resilience – overwhelm

- CHEERFULNESS, gaiety, happiness.
- EXCITEMENT, excitable; Ailments from, aggravates; mental and emotional consequences of.
- CARES, worries, full of; Aggravates, ailments from.
- SLEEPLESSNESS; Perspiration; with (62).

Suppression of emotions – Sublimation of libido

Male

- EMISSIONS, pollutions, seminal; frequent; old men, in (6): **Agn.**, aq-kron., bar-c., caust., nat-c., sulph.
- EMISSIONS, pollutions, seminal; old men, in (8): **Agn.**, aq-kron., *bar-c.*, brom., caust., *nat-c.*, staph., *sulph.*

Exhaustion – mental and physical

Perspiration

- COLD; Exertion of body or mind, after slight (6): act-sp., aq-kron., **Calc.**, cocc., **HEP.**, **SEP.**

Generalities

- WEAKNESS; menses; during; lie down, desire to (6): apoc., aq-kron., bell., carb-an., ip., **Nit-ac.**
- WEAKNESS; extreme; menses, after (24): **Alum.**, am-c., am-m., aq-kron., **Ars.**, calc., **Carb-an.**, carb-v., **Chin.**, cimic., **Cocc.**, ferr., glyc., graph., iod., ip., kali-c., mag-c., phos., thlaspi, **Tril.**, *tub.*, **Verat.**, vinc.

Clinical Rubric Clusters

Chorea

Extremities

- MOTION, motions; rotation; lower limbs (1): aq-kron.
- MOTION, motions; rotation (5): alum., aq-kron., bell., cann-i., **Stram.**

Generalities

- MOTION, motions; rotations (7): alum., aq-kron., bell., **Camph.**, cann-i., cann-s., **Stram.**

Trembling, weakness, paralysis and oedema lower limbs

- PAIN; Undulating, waving (18); lying, while (1): aq-kron.
- PARALYSIS; Lower limbs.
- TREMBLING; Lower limbs; knees,
- SWELLING****: Oedematous, dropsical.

Menstrual disorders -Tendency to miscarry

- MENSES; Late, too; girls, young (19): Acon., Apis, aq-kron., CALC., calc-p., **Caust.**, Cocc., cupr., **Ferr.**, **Graph.**, **Kali-c.**, **Nat-m.**, **Petr.**, PULS., SABIN., senec., **Sep.**, spig., SULPH., **Verat.**
- MENSES; Absent, amenorrhea.
- MENSES; Profuse; Protracted, prolonged.

- ABORTION; Tendency to ATONY; Uterus, inertia uteri.

Anaemia

Heart, circulation

- PALPITATION heart; Anaemia; from (16): aq-kron., ars., **Carb-v.**, **Chin.**, **Crat.**, dig., **Ferr.**, kali-c., kali-fcy., nat-m., **Ph-ac.**, **Phos.**, Puls., **Sep.**, spig., trinit., verat.

Head

- PAIN, headache; anaemia, with (23): *anag.*, aq-kron., ars., **Calc-p.**, camph-br., **Chin.**, chin-ar., cina, coca, **Cycl.**, eucal., **Ferr.**, **Ferr-p.**, kalm., lac-d., **Nat-m.**, nux-v., **Ph-ac.**, sang., **Senec.**, sulph., trinit., ZINC.

Female

- MENSES; suppressed; anaemia, in (32): **Alum.**, aq-kron., ars., ars-i., **Calc.**, caust., chin., cocc., coch., con., cupr., cycl., **Ferr.**, ferr-ar., goss., **Graph.**, **Helon.**, iod., **Kali-c.**, kali-ma., kali-p., kron., mag-acet., nat-c., **Nat-m.**, ovi-g-p., **Puls.**, rub-t., **Senec.**, **Sep.**, **Sin-n.**, sulph., xan.

Extremities

- COLDNESS, chilliness; sensation of; lower limbs; warm to touch, yet (9): aq-kron., **Coloc.**, dig., gink., **Ign.**, phos., polyg., **Sulph.**, ther.
- PAIN; undulating, waving; lower limbs (21): aego-p., anac., aq-kron., arn., asaf., bamb-a., clem., cocc., ign., kron., lappa, led., lyc., mez., olnd., ph-ac., plat., rhod., sep., *sul-ac.*, ulm-c., zing.

Generalities

- COLDNESS, lack of vital heat; touch, though warm to the (14): aq-kron., **Coloc.**, corn., dig., gink., haliae-lc., **Ign.**, m-aust., phos., polyg., psor., **Sulph.**, ther., zinc-m.
- DISCHARGES, secretions; Ameliorate; Suppressed aggravates.

AQUA LANDECK

Source

A spring rising at Landeck in the Tyrol in Germany.

Contents

The analysis of contents of the spring has been lost. The town still exists but is not a spa.

Rubrics

Sensitivity and vulnerability: emotional and cognitive – loss of resilience – overwhelm

Eyes

- AMBLYOPIA; excitement, strong emotional, aggravates (2): ant-t., aq-land.
- Excitement, excitable; ailments from, aggravates.

Clinical Rubric Clusters

Head Injuries with concussion and neurological damage – paralysis, convulsions and dilated or fixed pupils or amblyopia (as supportive treatment)

Compare with: Arnica montana, Artemisia vulgaris, Hypericum, Cicuta virosa, Natrum sulphuricum.

Generalities

- CONVULSIONS, spasms; Concussion of brain, after (12): absin., aq-land., **ARN.**, Art-v., **CIC.**, **Cupr.**, hell., hyos., **Hyper.**, **Led.**, meli., **Nat-s.**

- CONVULSIONS, spasms; Injuries, from; head, of (15): absin., aq-land., **ARN.**, **Art-v.**, bufo, **CIC.**, **Cupr.**, hell., hyos., **Hyper.**, **Led.**, meli., **Nat-s.**, **OENA.**, sol-c.

Generalities; PARALYSIS:

- PARALYSIS; spinal complaints, in (28): alum., aq-land., arn., ars., **Calc.**, **Cocc.**, dinitrob., diph., form., **Gels.**, **Hyper.**, *kali-p.*, karw-h., kres., lachn., land., lat-m., **Lath.**, mang., **Med.**, **Nat-m.**, **Nux-v.**, phos., **Plb.**, plect., **Sec.**, **Sil.**, ust., **Zinc.**

Eyes

- Amblyopia, dilatation; pupils, mydriasis fixed, pupils.

Gout

- Extremities; PAIN; gouty; toes (59); first (51).
- Generalities; PAIN; joints, articulations pain; gouty.

AQUA LIPPSPRINGE

Source

The water of the mineral spring in Lippspringe, Westphalia, Germany.

Contents

Contains mainly sodium sulphate, magnesium sulphate, calcium sulphate, calcium chloride plus carbonic acid, nitrogen and oxygen gases.

- Row 2: Carbonic acid, nitrogen and oxygen gases.
- Row 3: Sodium sulphate, magnesium sulphate.
- Row 4: Calcium sulphate calcium chloride.

Rubrics

Sensitivity and vulnerability: emotional and cognitive – loss of resilience – overwhelm

- COMFORT, sensation of; urination, after (1): aq-lipp.

- WRITING; Desire for (7): aq-lipp., *arist-cl.*, chin., diox., gels., hura, irid., psor., sphing., **Stram**.

DREAMS: Children

- Child; lying; on ice, her little child, she feared it would fall into water (1): aq-lipp.
- Water; falling into; child, her (3): aq-lipp., eupi., nitro.

DREAMS; horses:

- Running; over her (1): aq-lipp.
- Running (3): aq-lipp., atro., *indg*.

Heart and Circulation

- PALPITATION heart; tumultuous, violent, vehement; evening (1): aq-lipp.
- PALPITATION heart; trembling, with; hands, of (6): acan-pl., am-c., aq-lipp., **Bov.**, elaps, thyr.

Sleep

- WAKING; Midnight; after; two a.m.; about; morning, until (1): aq-lipp.

Suppression of Emotions – Sublimation of libido

Female

- PAIN; Rubbing aggravates (1): aq-lipp.
- PAIN; burning, smarting; rub, must (2): aq-lipp., **KREOS**.

Abdomen

- TINGLING, prickling; spleen region (2): aq-lipp., ruta.
- TINGLING, prickling; hypochondria (4): aq-lipp., **Ip.**, ruta, solid.

Rectum

- ITCHING; rubbing; ameliorates (3): aq-lipp., sac-l., ser-ang.

Exhaustion – mind and body

Extremities

- HEAVINESS, weariness; feet; walking; after; short (1): aq-lipp.
- HEAVINESS, weariness; feet; walking; after (10): alum., aq-lipp., **Arn.**, art-v., cann-s., caust., **Con.**, murx., **Rhus-t.**, ruta.

Clinical Rubric Clusters

Rheumatic Disorders

Back

- PAIN; drawing; cervical region; headache, during (1): aq-lipp.
- PAIN; lumbar region, lumbago; night; lying on left side (2): aq-lipp., bamb-a.

Sleep

- WAKING; pain, from; back, in (12): ang., aq-lipp., **Bry.**, carc., chion., cinis-p., helo., holm., hom., hydr., plut-n., sel.

Extremities

- PAIN; paralytic; legs; bones, tibia; walking aggravates (1): aq-lipp.
- PAIN; paralytic; legs; bones, tibia (7): aq-lipp., arg., card-m., cycl., *eug.*, mez., petr.
- PAIN; paralytic; bones; long (12): aq-lipp., arg., **Calc.**, card-m., caust., cham., cycl., eug., mez., nit-ac., petr., phos.
- PAIN; stitching; knees; extending to; ankles (4): aq-lipp., **Cham.**, scroph-n., stel.

Irritable bowel syndrome

Stomach

- DISORDERED; grapes, sour, aggravates (1): aq-lipp.
- PAIN; lying; aggravates; back, on (6): alumn., aq-lipp., **Carb-v.**, *caust.*, lac-del., **Lyc.**
- PAIN; lying; ameliorates; side, on (9): aq-lipp., **Chel.**, **Lyc.**, mag-m., merc., neod., plac., sang., squil.
- PAIN; pressing; lying; ameliorates; side, on (1): aq-lipp.
- PAIN; pressing; lying; ameliorates (7): ambr., aq-lipp., calc., chin., **Graph.**, lyc., stront-c.
- VOMITING; chilliness, with (14): aeth., aq-lipp., arn., ars., corn-a., dulc., hyosin., kali-br., *lyc.*, merc-cy., puls., tab., **Verat.**, vip.
- VOMITING; mucous; sour (11): aq-lipp., arn., *bor.*, **Chin.**, jab., **Kali-bi.**, **Kali-c.**, **Nat-s.**, **NUX-V.**, *verat.*, zinc-acet.

Abdomen

- PAIN; sudden, paroxysmal; vomiting, with (1): aq-lipp.
- PAIN; cramping, gripping; stool, as before (7): aphis., aq-lipp., chel., mang., raph., sin-a., **Trom.**

Rectum

- URGING, desire; rising; aggravates (6): **Aloe**, aq-lipp., croto-t., nat-ox., rheum, rumx.

Stool

- SHEEP dung, like; morning (1): aq-lipp.

Skin Eruptions: bright red with areola

Violent itching, must scratch, much worse bathing – compare Sulphur.

Skin

- ERUPTIONS; itching; evening; bed, in (3): aq-lipp., *merc-pr-a.*, oxpr.
- Merc-pr-a = Mercurius precuipitatus albus; oxpr. = Oxpranolol).
- ERUPTIONS; itching; bathing, washing; aggravates (8): aq-lipp., **Clem.**, coriand., germ., lappa, mez., **Rhus-v.**, sulph.
- ERUPTIONS; pimples; areola, with (9): aloe, aq-lipp., berb., bor., gels., hema-h., morph., nat-m., tarent-c.
- ERUPTIONS; rash; scarlatina, after (7): **Ail.**, apis, aq-lipp., **Bell.**, phyt., rhus-t., sulph.

Abdomen

- ERUPTIONS; pimples; red; areola, with (2): aloe, aq-lipp.
- ERUPTIONS; pimples; itching (9): aloe, aq-lipp., bry., dulc., lac-v-b., lsd, nat-c., **Staph.**, tell.

Ears

- ITCHING; scratching; must (7): agav-t., alum., aq-lipp., **Arg.**, arist-cl., *mosch.*, nat-p.

Nose

- ITCHING, tickling; violent (16): aq-lipp., *arg-n.*, **Coc-c.**, *coloc.*, eug., hell-v., lyc., mag-c., *merc.*, morph-s., *mur-ac.*, nat-c., nat-p., *nit-ac.*, peti.

Tickling Cough (Compare Coccus cacti)

Sleep

- WAKING; tickling in larynx, from (2): aq-lipp., **COC-C.**

Cough

- DRY; tickling, from; throat, in (10): *am-m.*, aq-lipp., aq-vichy-g., crot-c., **Kali-c.**, **Phos.**, plut-n., sang., sid-al., zinc-i.

Larynx and Trachea

- TICKLING in air passages; waking, on (4): aq-lipp., carb-v., cetr., ham.
- MUCOUS in air passages; tenacious; trachea (7): aq-lipp., aq-tep., **Bry.**, **Cann-s.**, just., **Nux-v.**, vinc.

Chest Pain – stitching – pleurisy – lobar pneumonia
(as supportive treatment)

- Worse: left side, deep inspiration sitting.
- Ameliorated by motion.

Chest

- PAIN; stitching; needles, as from; sides (1): aq-lipp.
- PAIN; stitching; sides; left; motion; ameliorates (1): aq-lipp.
- PAIN; stitching; sides; left; inspiration aggravates; deep (6): aq-lipp., **Bry.**, com., **KALI-C.**, ther., *valer.*
- PAIN; sides; left; motion; ameliorates (2): aq-lipp., hydr-ac.
- PAIN; sides; left; sitting aggravates (7): anac., aq-lipp. arg., atista, dulc., kali-i., rhus-t.

Tuberculosis – pulmonary with haemoptysis – left lung worst
with pleurisy – bleeding from lungs alternating with bleeding
from rectum – as supportive treatment

Chest

- PAIN; compressing; lungs (5): abies-n., aq-lipp. bapt., cina, dig.
- HEAVINESS; walking aggravates (7): am-m., aq-lipp., dys-co., lact., merc., muc-nas., *phos.*

Expectoration

- BLOODY, spitting of blood; alternating with; stool, bloody (1): aq-lipp.
- BLOODY, spitting of blood; morning; rising, on or after (5): aesc., alumn., aq-lipp., **Ferr.**, ferr-acet.
- BLOODY, spitting of blood; thin (18): acal., aq-lipp., carb-an., carb-v., dig., ferr., ferr-p., **GELS.**, graph., kreos., laur., merc., nux-m., puls., **SABIN.**, sec., stram., sul-ac.
- WHITE; egg, of, like (12): agav-t., aq-lipp., **Arn.**, benz., *crat.*, linu-c., **NAT-M.**, **Nat-s.**, sang., still., **Verat-v.**, visc.

Stool

- BLOODY; alternating with haemoptysis (1): aq-lipp.

Useful or Unusual Rubrics

Vertigo

- STANDING; ameliorates; still (1): aq-lipp.
- STANDING; ameliorates (5): aq-lipp., calc., nat-glut., nux-v., phos.

Head

- PAIN, headache; drawing; vertex; right (2): aq-lipp., *spig.*
- PAIN, headache; stitching; vertex; right (7): aq-lipp., electr., lith-c., mag-m., olea, olnd., toxop-p.

Vision

- FLICKERING; reading, from; stooped (1): aq-lipp.
- FLICKERING; stooping aggravates (2): aq-lipp., bell.
- FLICKERING; reading, from (14): *aq-carl.*, aq-lipp., aran., arn., *bell.*, cob., **Cycl.**, hell-f., *lach.*, merc., *merl.*, onc-t., *ph-ac.*, **Seneg.**

Face

- HEAT; glowing (14): *acon.*, aq-lipp., astac., aza., *bell.*, *carb-v.*, *croc.*, *gran.*, inul., *nux-v.*, *phos.*, plat., rham-cal., *tab.*

Throat

- DRYNESS: sugar ameliorates (1): aq-lipp.
- ROUGHNESS, scraping sensation; mucus, with; throat, in (8): amyg-am., aq-lipp., *calc.*, *mag-m.*, muc-nas., parth., por-m., **Rhod.**

Abdomen

- TINGLING, prickling (15): aq-lipp., cerv., gins., **Ip.**, kreos., loxo-r., mag-m., mur-ac., petr., **Plat.**, ruta, solid., tax., verat., zinc.

Rectum

- PROLAPSE; lying down aggravates (1): aq-lipp.
- ITCHING; leucorrhoea, with (2): aq-lipp., dict.
- HAEMORRHOIDS; stitching; stool, during (2): aq-lipp., meteo-a.
- PAIN; tenesmus, painful urging; morning; rising, after (2): aeth., aq-lipp.
- PAIN; tenesmus, painful urging; morning (5): aeth., aq-lipp., kali-bi., nicc., tub.

- HAEMORRHAGE: thin, fluid, does not coagulate (8): aq-lipp., **Ars.**, **Carb-v.**, chlor., **CROT-H.**, **Lach.**, **Nit-ac.**, **Phos.**

⚠ **This symptom requires referral for thorough medical unves-tigation until a clear diagnosis is made.**

Bladder

- URGING to urinate, morbid desire; rising, on (9): aloe, ambr., aq-lipp., berb., carb-v., mez., nat-p., plan., **SULPH.**

Male

- SMEGMA increased; thin (1): aq-lipp.
- SMEGMA increased (12): *alum.*, aq-lipp., bry., **Canth.**, **CAUST.**, hema-h., lach., *nat-c.*, **Nux-v.**, **Sang.**, **Sulph.**, **Sumb.**

Female

- LEUCORRHOEA; bloody; mucous (7): aloe, aq-lipp., bar-c., *carb-v.*, merc-c., sep., sul-ac.
- PAIN; sore, bruised; walking aggravates (6): **Apis**, aq-lipp., **ARN.**, **BRY.**, fago., **Lac-c.**

Chest

- HEAVINESS; coition, after (1): aq-lipp.
- HEAVINESS: smoking aggravates (1): aq-lipp.
- PERSPIRATION; morning (9): aq-lipp., bamb-a., **Bov.**, **Cocc.**, graph., kali-n., lsd, sep., tub.

Extremities

- CRAMPS; legs; calves; evening (14): aq-lipp., **Ars.**, bell., berb., carb-v., kali-n., mag-c., nit-ac., nux-m., nux-v., **Puls.**, sel., **Sil.**, sulph.

Generalities

- HEAT; flushes of; loosening clothes ameliorates (2): aq-lipp., nicc-s.
- FOOD and drinks; grapes; aggravates (6): aq-lipp., chin., chir-f., ox-ac., verat., viol-o.

Vision

- FLICKERING; reading, from (14): *aq-carl.*, aq-lipp., aran., arn., *bell.*, cob., **Cycl.**, hell-f., *lach.*, merc., *merl.*, onc-t., *ph-ac.*, **Seneg.**

Compare Related Remedies

Aqua – comprising: Aqua Carlsbad, Aqua Teplitz, Aqua Vichy Grande Grille

Related level: Share and Compare Rubrics (too few to make a cluster).

Vision

- FLICKERING; reading, from (14): *aq-carl.*, aq-lipp., aran., arn., *bell.*, cob., **Cycl.**, hell-f., *lach.*, merc., *merl.*, onc-t., *ph-ac.*, **Seneg.**

Larynx trachea

- MUCOUS in air passages; tenacious; trachea (7): aq-lipp., aq-tep., **Bry.**, **Cann-s.**, just., **Nux-v.**, vinc.

Cough

- DRY; tickling, from; throat, in (10): *am-m.*, aq-lipp., aq-vichy-g., crot-c., **Kali-c.**, **Phos.**, plut-n., sang., sid-al., zinc-i.

Sulphur

Related level: Clinical Rubric Clusters.

Back

- PAIN; lumbar region, lumbago; lying; aggravates; side, on; left (4): agar., aq-lipp., bamb-a., **SULPH.**

Bladder

- URGING to urinate, morbid desire; morning; rising, on or after (6): ambr., aq-lipp., berb., mez., plan., **SULPH.**

Female

- PAIN; sore, bruised; leucorrhoea, from (7): aq-lipp., calc., **Carb-v.**, ferr., kreos., rob., **Sulph.**

Argentum metallicum, Chrysarobinum

Related level: Clinical Rubric Clusters.

Skin

- ITCHING; scratching; must (7): agav-t., alum., aq-lipp., **Arg.**, arist-cl., *mosch.*, nat-p.

Ears

- ITCHING; Violent (11): agar., alum., aq-lipp., **Arg.**, arist-cl., *calc.*, *carb-v.*, **CHRYSAR.**, *con.*, *kali-c.*, *kali-n.*, nat-p., *phos.*, psor., *sep.*, *sulph.*, thuj., *tong.*

Milks – Lac caninum, Lac delphinium, Lac vaccini flos

Related level: Clinical Rubric Clusters.

Female

- PAIN; sore, bruised; walking aggravates (6): **Apis**, aq-lipp., **ARN.**, **BRY.**, fago., **Lac-c.**

Stomach

- PAIN; lying; aggravates; back, on (6): alumn., aq-lipp., **Carb-v.**, *caust.*, lac-del., **Lyc.**

DREAMS

- Coffins (12): anac., aq-lipp., *brom.*, form., ignis, lac-v-f., lat-h., lepi., mand., merc-i-f., tax., vip.

AQUA MEINBERG PYRMONT

Source

Water mixed from 2 cold springs rising 20km apart in Bad Meinberg and Bad Pyrmont in Germany.

Content

The analysis of contents of the springs has been lost. The towns still exists but neither is a spa.

Rubrics

Paralysis – Compare Causticum and Manganum

Face

- PARALYSIS; right (17): aq-mein., **Arn.**, bell., butho-t., cadm-s., **Caust.**, hep., kali-chl., kali-m., kali-p., methylp-h., ol-an., **Phos.**, plb., sil., tela, zinc-p.

Mouth

- PARALYSIS; tongue; right (2): aq-mein., bell.
- SALIVATION; paralysis; with (4): abel., aq-mein., cyrt-p., **Mang.**

- Generalities; PARALYSIS; right (67).
- Speech and Voice; DIFFICULT speech; paralysis of organs, from (53).

Trigeminal Neuralgia on right

- Face; PAIN; neuralgic, prosopalgia; right (39).
- Face; PAIN; motion; aggravates; muscles of face, of (101).

Generalities

- PAIN; neuralgic; right (99).

Compare Nosodes in Recurrent Tonsilitis

Streptococccinum, DPT, Diphtherinum, Diphtherotoxinum, Dysentery co. (Bach), Morgan Pure, Morgan Gaertner, Sycotic Co. (Paterson), Psorinum, Tuberculinum bovinum.

Throat

- INFLAMMATION, sore throat; recurrent, tonsils (40): **Ail.**, **Alumn.**, aq-mein., aur-m-n., **BAR-C.**, **Bar-m.**, bufo, calc., carc., diph., diphtox., dpt, dys-co., ferr., guai., **Hep.**, kali-i., kali-m., lach., lyc., morg., morg-g., neod-f., **Nit-ac.**, phos., phyt., pitu-a., plut-n., **PSOR.**, sama-m., **Sang.**, sep., **Sil.**, **STREPT.**, sulph., syc-co., thal., thymin., **TUB.**, vesp.

AQUA TUNBRIDGE WELLS

Source

The spring water has been used medicinally since Roman times. Royal Tunbridge Wells, Kent, England became a popular and very fashionable spa town in the 17th and 18th centuries with Royal patronage.

Content

Mainly potassium and iron (ferrous) salts.

Proving

Two provings[4]

- A meditative proving by staff of Helios Pharmacy Tunbridge Wells after potentising the water to 40C.
- Students of the Guild of Homeopaths in 1997 took 6C without being aware what the remedy was.

Rubrics

Scholten's row and column themes:[5]

Row 4 themes:

- Duty, work, task, craft – able, useful, practical.
- Be an adult and earn your rightful place in the village community.
- Official control.
- Observed, criticised; failure, guilt, crime, persecuted, tried.

Column 1 themes:

- Begin, start, initiate.
- Impulsive, instinctive, spontaneous, unpredictable.
- One, single, single-minded, unreflective, thoughtless, fool.
- Simple, simpleton, naive, childish.

Column 8 themes:

- Build, construct, calculate, plan, deadline.
- Force, pressure, push through hard, struggle on, onwards.
- Persevere, endurance.
- Compress, heavy, resistance, opposition, oppression.

Social Conformity with Fear of Being Judged

- Strong desire to conform to the rules.
- Fastidious in observing regulations guidelines.
- Embarrassed uncomfortable if seen to be breaking the rules.
- Adhering to the rules gives a sense of structure they otherwise lack.
- Sensation of being observed (similar to *Aqua marina*).

Suppression of emotions – Sublimation of libido

- Present a proper correct mask of politeness which can deceive.
- Conceal whatever is ugly or considered unnatural.
- Eventually can be cut off from their true emotions and yet lost in self-disgust, self loathing, desolation and grief.
- Prefers to be alone, actively seek anonymity.
- Long sufferance in silence and hopelessness.
- Cannot make friends easily or does so only with those very similar to themselves – or become carers for the very ill or very handicapped.
- Fear of intimate relationships – men can feel intimidated by women.
- Too difficult to change or get better – would entail dealing with issues too awful to contemplate.

Repression and schism – a separation impossible to bridge

- Between generations.
- Between self and others.
- Between parent and child.
- Rebellious polarity – strong desire to break the rules – to indulge in an affair – and infuriate the family.

- Sensation of isolation – as if separated from society or separated from friends or even making friends.
- Feels outcast even unable to make eye contact with others – ashamed of oneself.
- Unresolved anger bitterness.
- Desolation crushed – hopelessness despair.
- Exhaustion – mental physical.

Clinical Rubric Clusters

During case taking, the mineral kingdom is clear, the themes of Row 4 are clear, Kali themes are clear plus there is something about Column 8 – it's hard, push through, never give in, plus something more that doesn't quite fit – a spiritual and intuitive side to the character – e.g. a gift for dowsing and a simple trust in that process.

Acne with scarring

Skin

- CICATRICES; eruptions, after (22): ant-c., aq-sanic., aq-tun., arg-n., art-v., *blatta*, brom., calc-ar., calc-sil., carb-an., caust., coenz-q., **Cop.**, **Kali-bi.**, **Kali-br.**, **Kali-i.**, mag-m., merc., mez., pip-n., sulph., thuj.

Face

- ERUPTIONS; acne; scars, leaving (17): ant-c., aq-tun., arg-n., art-v., brom., calc-ar., calc-sil., carb-an., caust., coenz-q., **Cop.**, **Kali-br.**, kali-i., mag-m., merc., sanic., thuj.

Heartburn, reflux, oesophagitis

- Heartburn water-brash with belching burning pain in oesophagus.
- Stomach feels heavy full – aggravated after drinking water or any liquids.
- Need to eat little infrequently.
- Much worse both from becoming too hungry or overeating.
- Desire for milk but milk aggravates.
- Hot water ameliorates but only for a short while.

Extreme nausea, vomiting

Supportive treatment during Cancer chemotherapy when Ipecac and/or Cadmium sulphuricum don't help.

Stomach

- VOMITING; cancer, in (37): acet-ac., act-sp., am-caust., ant-c., aq-tun., arg-n., **Ars.**, art-v., bism., **Cadm-s.**, calen., **Carb-ac.**, **Carb-an.**, **Con.**, crot-h., cund., cupr-acet., eucal., graph., hydr., ip., iris, kali-bi., *kreos.*, lach., lyc., mag-c., mag-p., merc., **Mez.**, nit-ac., orni., **Phos.**, phyt., rob., sul-ac., verat-v.

Other Useful Symptoms

- Thick sputum deep within lungs – difficult to hawk up – painful cough which aggravates gastro-intestinal symptoms.
- Eczema of external genitals – sore red scaly itching – skin red and swollen.
- Genital herpetic eruptions.
- Menses clotted smell rotten.

Compare/Related Remedies
Carbo animalis and Kali salt.

AQUA VOESLAU

Source

A mineral spring rising at the spa town of Bad Voeslau in Austria – remedy made from the fresh water.

Contents

The water contains:

- Row 3: Magnesium carbonate, magnesium sulphate, magnesium chloride, sodium sulphate, sodium chloride, alumina and silica.
- Row 4: Calcium carbonate, calcium sulphate, calcium chloride, ferrous nitrate.

Rubrics

Sensitivity and vulnerability: emotional and cognitive – loss of resilience – overwhelm

- RESTLESSNESS, nervousness; work, during (9): aq-voes., bamb-a., cit-a., cortico., **GRAPH.**, hep., kola., neod-o., onos.
- RESTLESSNESS, nervousness; excitable (21): **Absin.**, aq-voes., asar., **CHAM.**, chin., diox., dysp-o., gink., **HYOS.**, **Ign.**, **Iod.**, kali-p., mand., myric., sabad., scut., **Sil.**, stram., **Teucr.**, zinc., zinc-val.

Stomach

- SENSITIVENESS; eating aggravates (2): aq-voes., kali-c.

Suppression of emotions – Sublimation of libido

Skin

- PAIN; biting; midnight, about (1): aq-voes.
- PAIN; biting; perspiration; before (1): aq-voes.

Male

- CONGESTION (10): achy., aq-voes., coloc., colocin., ham., lac-v-b., lycps., med., merc-s., yohim.

Sleep

- SLEEPINESS; overpowering; afternoon (14): aq-voes., bruc., croto-t., *excr-can.*, hydr., hyos., kali-c., lyc., nat-c., pall., **PULS.**, *staph.*, stel., tax.

Clinical Rubric Clusters

Skin – Urticaria

- ERUPTIONS; urticaria, nettle-rash; desquamation, with (1): aq-voes.
- ERUPTIONS; urticaria, nettle-rash; itching; with (31).

Liver

Abdomen

- TENSION; liver region; extending to right shoulder (1): aq-voes.
- PAIN; pressing; liver; extending to; shoulder, right (1): aq-voes.
- PAIN; liver; extending to; shoulder; right (15): aq-voes., bamb-a., **Bry.**, **Card-m.**, chel., crot-h., harp., **Kali-bi.**, kali-c., **Med.**, merc-c., rhus-t., **SEP.**, thuj., vip.

Useful or Unusual rubrics

Face

- HEAT; flushes; thirst, without, thirstless (2): aq-voes, *thuj.*

Throat

- PAIN; food; warm; aggravates (4): aq-voes., canth., kali-c., merc-c.

Stomach

- SENSITIVENESS; eating aggravates (2): aq-voes., kali-c.

AQUA WEILBACH

Source

Water from the Dreirohrenbrunnen spring rises from three spouts into a sandstone trough in the town of Weilbach in Bavaria, Germany.

Content

The analysis of contents of the spring has been lost. The town still exists but is not a spa.

Rubrics

Sensitivity and vulnerability: emotional and cognitive – loss of resilience – overwhelm

Heart and circulation

- PULSE, heartbeat; febrile (22): **Acon.**, alum., alumn., anthro., aq-kiss., aq-weil., **Ars.**, **Bell.**, bov., croc., gins., lac-ac., merc-c., mez., morph., plb., sars., sec., **Stram.**, **Sulph.**, thuj., vip.
- EXCITEMENT, excitable; Ailments from, aggravates.

Clinical

Urinary tract infection

- URINATION; difficult, dysuria; night (7): ant-c., aq-weil., **Cic.**, hydrc., **Merc.**, **Solid.**, *spig.*

- INFLAMMATION Catarrhal.
- PAIN; Urination; during URINATION; Frequent.

Urine

- CLOUDY SEDIMENT; Purulent.
- OFFENSIVE STRONG odour THICK.

Mercury toxicity

- Generalities; INTOXICATION, after; Mercury.
- Face; BLACK and EARTHY and GRAYISH.
- Skin; DRYNESS and BLACKISH and GRAY.

Syphilis

- Generalities; SYPHILIS.
- Generalities; NIGHT, nine pm. – five am. Aggravates.
- Extremities; PAIN; **Lower limbs*****; Legs; bones; tibia.

AQUA WIESBADEN

Source

The spring at Wiesbaden, west of Frankfurt in Germany has been used medicinally for many centuries. The spa town continues to be popular.

Content

- Row 2: Carbonic acid, nitrogen, lithium chloride, ammonium chloride.
- Row 3: Sodium chloride, magnesium chloride, magnesium bromide, magnesium carbonate, magnesium iodate, aluminium silicate.
- Row 4: Potassium chloride, calcium chloride, calcium carbonate, calcium arsenate, calcium phosphate, calcium sulphate, ferrous carbonate, manganese carbonate, copper carbonate.
- Row 5: Strontium carbonicum.

Related bowel nosodes – Morgan Pure, Sycotic Co.

Compare: Stramonium, Belladonna, Graphites.

Rubrics

Sensitivity and vulnerability: emotional and cognitive – loss of resilience – overwhelm

- GESTURES, makes; Light (5): aq-wies., chin., clem., coff., phel.
- Generalities; ENERGY, lots of STRENGTH; Sensation of.
- ACTIVITY CHEERFULNESS, gaiety, happiness.

Generalities

- CLOTHING; Intolerance of, loosening ameliorates.

Chest

- PRESSURE; Aggravates; clothes, of.

Respiration

- DIFFICULT; Clothing aggravates.
- LOOSENING clothes ameliorates.

Suppression of emotions – Sublimation of libido

Heart and Circulation

- ORGASM of blood; sleep; during (2): ang., aq-wies.
- PULSE, heartbeat; rapid, tachycardia; violent (5): aq-wies., bry., dig., ferr-i., nux-m.

Chest

- CONSTRICTION: clothes, must loosen (4): aq-wies., eupi., salv., xan.

Head

- ITCHING; incessant (1); aq-wies.

Stomach

- HICCOUGH; menses, during (1): aq-wies.

Abdomen

- CONSTRICTION; diaphragm (15): aq-wies., arn., **Asar.**, cact., canth., cench., cupr-acet., hydr-ac., kali-cy., lepi., lyc., merc-i-r., mez., **Nux-v.**, tarax.

Exhaustion – mind and body

Generalities

- WEAKNESS; perspiration; ameliorates (1): aq-wies.

- WEARINESS; morning; bed, in (17): alum., berb., aq-wies., canth., carb-an., chin., con., erig., lact., loxo-r., lyc., mag-c., *petr.*, phos., **Staph.**, teg-a., teucr.

Water and Thirst

- CRAMPS; Muscles; water, approaching (1): aq-wies.
- CONVULSIONS, spasms; water; aversion (2): aq-wies., stram.
- CONVULSIONS, spasms; water; sight of, at (10): anan., aq-wies., *ars.*, **Bell., CANTH., Hyos., LYSS., STRAM.**, tanac., ter.
- FOOD drinks; Drinks; desires thirst, without, thirstless (17): aeth., **Ang.**, aq-wies., **Ars.**, bell., **Calad., Camph., Cimx.**, *cocc.*, **Coloc.**, graph., *nux-m.*, nux-v., ph-ac., phos., **Rhus-t.**, samb.

Clinical Rubric Clusters

Hernia – actual femoral and sensation as if inguinal

Abdomen

- HERNIA; femoral (3): **Aq-Wies.**, ferr-pic., nux-v.

Extremities

- PAIN; hernia would appear, as if; hips (1): aq-wies.
- HERNIA; Sensation of, inguinal region (14): **Alum.**, aq-wies., calc-ar., dig., iris-foe., kali-bi., lyc., rhus-r., *rhus-t.*, sarcol-ac., sel., sep., sul-ac., ter.

Abdomen

- PAIN; pressing; protrude, as if something would (5): aq-wies., clem., nit-ac., petr., **SEP.**

Inflammatory arthritis and Gout

Extremities

- PAIN; rheumatic; thighs; walking aggravates (2): aq-wies., daph.
- PAIN; rheumatic; lower limbs; walking aggravates (7): aq-wies., *carc.*, daph., jug-r., kali-bi., nat-m., sumb.
- PAIN; rheumatic; thighs; right (5): aq-wies., cass., caust., colch., sang.

- SWELLING; hot; knees (9): aq-wies., **Bell., Calc., Chin., Ferr-p., Iod., PULS.**, stict., **VERAT-V.**
- SWELLING; hot; joints (17): act-sp., aq-wies., ars., **Bell., Bry., Calc., Chin., Ferr-p., Hep., Iod.**, kali-c., **Led.**, med., **MERC., PULS.**, stict., **VERAT-V.**
- SWELLING; knees; left (12): adam., **Aesc.**, aq-wies., bac., benz-ac., **Cic.**, colch., coloc., lyc., merc-succ., sapin., sulph.

- SWELLING; hands; perspiration ameliorates (2): aq-wies., hist.
- SWELLING; feet; perspiration; ameliorates (1): aq-wies.
- FELON, onychia, paronychia; tendons (18): all-c., anthr., **Apis**, **Aq-Wies**, bufo, graph., **Hep.**, **Lach.**, **Led.**, **Merc.**, nat-s., **Nit-ac.**, ran-b., rhus-t., **SIL.**, sulph., **Syph.**, **Thlaspi.**

Hearing

- IMPAIRED; rheumatic, gouty diathesis (17): aq-wies., calc., calc-p., ferr., **Ferr-pic.**, guai., ham., kali-i., led., mang., merc., **Petr.**, rhod., rhus-t., sil., sulph., **Visc.**

Rapid Growth of Scalp Hair which can become darker

Head

- DARKER, hair becomes (5): **Aq-Wies.**, aq-wild., chloram., jab., piloc.
- GROWTH; Hair, of, increased (9): all-c., **Aq-Wies.**, electr., gink., lyc., mez., phyt., **Sac-alb.**, *thuj.*
- HARD; hair (2): aq-wies., **Thuj.**
- BRITTLE; Hair (14): aq-wies., ars., bell., **Bor.**, dys-co., **Fl-ac.**, graph., harp., **Kali-c.**, lyc., **Psor.**, sals-t., *thuj.*, toxop-p.

Corns callosities and Cracked heels

Extremities

- CORNS; drop off (1): aq-wies.
- CORNS; elevated (1): aq-wies.
- CORNS; soft (2): aq-wies., **Sil.**
- CORNS; soft; toes, between (2): aq-wies., sil.

- CALLOSITIES, horny; Hands (17): **Am-c.**, ant-c., aq-wies., bor., calc-f., cist., gast., **GRAPH.**, kali-ar., merc-i-r., nat-m., **Phos.**, posit., rhus-v., sil., **SULPH.**, thuj.
- CRACKS, fissures; Feet; heels (34): acon., aq-wies., **Ars.**, arund., aur., bac., bani-c., c-di-o., calc., calc-f., coc-c., erb-c., fic-mac., **Kali-c.**, kali-p., lach., **Lyc.**, merc., **Morg.**, **Nat-m.**, onc-t., oryc-c., pyrit., rauw., rib-ac., sars., **SEP.**, sil., staph., stram., **Sulph.**, **Syc-co.**, thul-c., til-c.

Earwax

- ITCHING; Wax, ameliorates after profuse discharge of (1): aq-wies.
- WAX altered; pale (2): aq-wies., **LACH.**
- WAX altered; mucous (3): aq-wies., cadm., con.
- WAX altered; soft (5): aq-wies., *kali-c.*, **Petr.**, sel., sil.

- WAX altered; hardened (11): **ALL-S.**, aq-wies., con., elaps, lach., **Mur-ac.**, **Petr.**, **PULS.**, sel., *semp.*, *verb.*
- WAX altered; flowing (15): am-m., anac., aq-wies., calc-s., helo., **Hep.**, **Kali-c.**, **Lyc.**, **Merc.**, mosch., **Nat-m.**, **Nit-ac.**, **Phos.**, **Puls.**, sel.
- WAX altered; thin (20): act-sp., *am-m.*, aq-wies., cadm., **Con.**, crot-h., flag-l., **Hep.**, iod., **Kali-c.**, lach., **Merc.**, mosch., **Petr.**, sel., **Sil.**, sulph., **Tell.**, tung., *zinc-o.*

Cramps

Extremities

- CRAMPS; thighs; menses; during (2): aq-wies., mag-m.
- CRAMPS; feet; menses, during (4): aq-wies., lachn., nicc., sulph.
- CRAMPS; menses; during (12): aq-wies., cimic., cupr., form., **Gels.**, **Graph.**, lachn., mag-m., nicc., phos., sulph., verat.

Other Unique Rubrics

Urine

- STIFFENING linen (1): **Aq-Wies.**
- SEDIMENT; yellow; green (1): aq-wies.

Vertigo

- TURNING in a circle, as if; menses, during (1): aq-wies.

Vision

- MOVING; objects seem to be; vertigo, in (1): aq-wies.

Face

- COBWEB sensation; left (1): aq-wies.
- PERSPIRATION; rub, must (1): aq-wies.

Mouth

- FOLDED skin; desquamating (1): aq-wies.
- SWELLING; tongue; under; blood-vessels (1): aq-wies.

Abdomen

- FERMENTATION; drinking aggravates (1): aq-wies.
- ITCHING; spots, in, on perspiration (1): aq-wies.
- PAIN; dragging, bearing down; extending; thighs, to; right (1): aq-wies.
- CONGESTION, hyperaemia; haemorrhage from anus ameliorates (1): aq-wies.

Stool

- BILIOUS; membranous, hardened (1): aq-wies.

Skin

- ITCHING; biting; salt, like (1): aq-wies.

Useful or Unusual Rubrics

Vision

- LOSS of vision, blindness; epistaxis; ameliorates (2): aq-wies., bell.

Stomach

- HICCOUGH; menses, during (1): aq-wies.
- HICCOUGH; cramps, with (4): aq-wies., carb-v., **Cupr-ar.**, *hyos.*

Female

- MENSES; profuse; climacteric period; after (1): aq-wies.

> ⚠ **This symptom requires referral to a gynaecologist for investigation to reach a clear diagnosis as it may be the presentation of uterine cancer.**

- MENSES; protracted, prolonged; fourteen days (5): aq-wies., card-m., Coloc., ust., **Xan.**

Sleep

- SLEEPINESS; morning; seven a.m. (3): aq-wies., calad., lac-h.
- SLEEPLESSNESS; heat; during; dry (7): aq-wies., **Caust.**, chin-s., clem., **Graph.**, nit-ac., **Thuj.**

Fever, heat

- ALTERNATING states; chill, with; menses, during (4): *am-c.*, aq-wies., sep., thuj.

Perspiration

- STAINING; parts affected (1): aq-wies.
- EGGS, like rotten (4): aq-wies., plb., **Staph.**, **Sulph.**

Skin

- ABSCESSES, suppurations; painful (4): aml-n., aq-wies., cyrt-p., nat-hchls.

- HARDNESS; parchment, like (24): *acon.*, aeth., aq-wies., **ARS.**, bac., **Calc-f.**, camph., **Chin.**, crot-h., *dig.*, dulc., *kali-c.*, led., **Lith-c.**, **Lyc.**, mag-c., op., **Petr.**, phos., rhus-t., sabad., **Sars.**, **Sil.**, *squil.*

Generalities

- STIFFNESS, rigidity; fractures, after (1): aq-wies.
- FOOD and drinks; refreshing things; desires; chill, during (2): aq-wies., cocc.
- HEAT; nausea, with (4): aq-wies., chel., lampr-s., naja-m.
- PAIN; burning, smarting; body, all over (4): apis, aq-wies., rad-br., stict.
- HAEMORRHAGE; ameliorates; anus, from (5): aesc., aq-tepo., aq-wies., calad., ovi-g-p.
- WOUNDS; gunshot, punctured (21): **APIS**, aq-wies., **Aran.**, **ARN.**, **Calen.**, **EUPHR.**, **Hyper.**, iod., **Lach.**, **Led.**, **NIT-AC.**, **Phase.**, plan., **PLB.**, **Puls.**, **Ruta**, staph., **SUL-AC.**, **Sulph.**, **Symph.**, urt-u.

Compare/Related Remedies
Compare/related at level of Clinical Rubric Clusters:

- Graphites and Petroleum – skin and wax and hearing.
- Solanaceae: Belladonna, Stramonium and Lyssinum.
- CONVULSIONS, spasms; water; sight of, at (10): anan., aq-wies., *ars.*, **Bell.**, **CANTH.**, **Hyos.**, **LYSS.**, **STRAM.**, tanac., ter.

Nosodes: Lyssinum, Syphilinum, Sycotic Co. Morgan Pure Paterson, Psorinum, Carcinosin, Bacillinum.

Aqua

Aqua Teplitz, Aqua Gastein, Aqua Carlsbad.

Generalities

- HAEMORRHAGE; ameliorates; anus, from (5): aesc., aq-tep., aq-wies., calad., ovi-g-p.

Extremities

- CALLOSITIES, horny; Hands (17): **Am-c.**, ant-c., aq-gast., aq-wies., bor., calc-f., cist., **GRAPH.**, kali-ar., merc-i-r., nat-m., **Phos.**, posit., rhus-v., sil., **SULPH.**, thuj.

Sleep

- DEEP; un-refreshing (22): alum., *aq-carl.*, aq-wies., blatta, chin-s., cinch., *conch.*, gink., lap-gr-m., **Mag-c.**, mel-alt., ost., **Pic-ac.**, psor., pter-a., rad-br., sal-ac., sarr., **Sol-m.**, stel., thuj., **Zinc.**

Acids

- Fluoric Acid, Muriatic Acid, Nitric Acid, Sarcolactic Acid, Sulphuric Acid and Benzoic Acid.

Compare/related at level of Clinical Rubric Clusters
Three rubric examples shown:

Extremities

- GROWTH; rapid, nails (11): aq-wies., calc., calc-f., falco-p., **FL-AC.**, hema-h., kali-i., ozone, *plac.*, thuj., ust.

Ears

- WAX altered; hardened (11): **ALL-S.**, aq-wies., con., elaps, lach., **Mur-ac.**, **Petr.**, **PULS.**, sel., *semp.*, verb.
- WAX altered; flowing (15): am-m., anac., aq-wies., calc-s., helo., **Hep.**, **Kali-c.**, **Lyc.**, **Merc.**, mosch., **Nat-m.**, **Nit-ac.**, **Phos.**, **Puls.**, sel.

AQUA WILDBAD

Source

Springs rising in the spa town of Wildbad, west of Stuttgart, Germany.

History

The Spa was mainly used for affections of the spinal cord – more than half the patients being paraplegic.

Content

- Row 2: Carbonic acid.
- Row 3: Sodium carbonate, sodium chloride, sodium sulphate, magnesium carbonate, alumina, silicic acid.
- Row 4: Potassium sulphate, calcium carbonate, ferrous carbonate and traces of manganese.

Proving

Proving of the water by Hartlaub and Kallenbach is referred to in some homeopathic books and websites, but the actual symptoms of the proving appear to be lost in the mists of time.[6]

Rubrics

Sensitivity and vulnerability: emotional and cognitive – loss of resilience – overwhelm

- EXCITEMENT, excitable; beer, after (2): aq-wild., coc-c.
- RESTLESSNESS, nervousness; midnight; after; four am. (5): aq-wild., clem., kreos., nit-ac., trom.

Face

- SENSITIVENESS; eyebrows (2): adam., aq-wild.

Head

- TENSION; scalp, external; forehead (4): anag., aq-wild., lycpr., *nit-ac.*

Sleep

- SLEEPLESSNESS; midnight; before; four am., until (13).
- SLEEPLESSNESS; midnight; after; four am., until (22).

Suppression of emotions – Sublimation of libido

Male

- ERECTIONS, troublesome; Painful; waking, on (1): aq-wild.
- PAIN; Spermatic cord; waking, on, after seminal emissions, pollutions (1): aq-wild.
- PAIN; Drawing; spermatic cord; waking, on, after seminal emissions, pollutions (1): aq-wild.

Perspiration

- WAKING; on or after; dreaming, after (7): am-c., anac., aq-wild., graph., meteo-a., neod., terb-o.

Face

- FORMICATION, crawling; mouth, about; left (1): aq-wild.
- FORMICATION, crawling; mouth, about (4): aq-wild., lap-laz., teg-a., toxop-p.
- FORMICATION, crawling; lips; lower (5): aq-wild., **Ars.**, bor., caust., sabad.
- TWITCHING; violent (3): aq-wild., cupr-ar., *phel.*

Exhaustion – mind and body

- Weakness with inclination to keep quiet – aggravated after walking.
- Weariness especially in the knees and ankles, so that he was frequently obliged to sit down.
- Sudden weariness after a walk; standing was so difficult that he was obliged to sit down; the ankles seemed loosened and not firm; on ascending a hill it seemed as though the joints of the knees and ankles would separate.
- Inclination to lie down, especially on the back to stretch out, with a feeling of comfort and warmth through the whole body.
- Aversion to business, especially after a bath.

Eyes

- PAIN; Evening; aggravates; writing, while (3): aq-wild., **Nat-m.**, sel.
- PAIN; Pressing; writing, while (3): *alum.*, aq-wild., con.

Extremities

- HEAVINESS, weariness; hips; exertion, slight, aggravates (1): aq-wild.
- HEAVINESS, weariness; knees; walking; after (5): aq-wild., berb., calc-s., ignis, ruta.
- HEAVINESS, weariness; ankles; walking aggravates (1): aq-wild.
- HEAVINESS, weariness; exertion, from (14).

Generalities

- WEAKNESS; sudden, paroxysmal; walking, from (4): aq-wild., carb-v., con.
- WEAKNESS; rest; ameliorates (12): achy., aq-wild., aran., atista, **BRY.**, gink., hydrog., mag-c., nat-m., nat-n., stann., uran-n.

Clinical Rubric Clusters

Hair becomes darker and hairy chin in women

Head

- DARKER, hair becomes (5): **Aq-Wies.**, aq-wild., chloram., jab., piloc.

Face

- HAIRY; chin; beard; darker than usual (1): aq-wild.
- HAIRY; chin; women, in (5): aq-wild., cer-c., geoc-c., ol-j., pall.

Paralysis after injuries

Generalities

- PARALYSIS; injuries, after (14): apoc., aq-wild., arn., bell., **Calc.**, con., cupr., hydr-ac., *hyper.*, kali-p., lath., **Led.**, **Op.**, staph.

Back

- CONCUSSION; spine (10): aq-wild., **Arn.**, **BELL-P.**, cic., con., euph-pu., fil., **HYPER.**, mez., phys.

Headaches

Head

- FULLNESS; lying, while (2): aq-wild., naja.
- HEAT; occiput; lying aggravates (1): *aq-wild.*
- PAIN, headache; pulsating, throbbing; occiput; night (2): aq-wild., **Lyc.**
- PAIN, headache; pulsating, throbbing; waking, on (5): aq-wild., ozone, *sia-c.*, sulph., tarent.
- PAIN, headache; pulsating, throbbing; night; aggravates (15): aq-wild., **Arg-n.**, bamb-a., bor., calc., calc-ar., camph., glon., helo., kreos., *m-aust.*, nux-m., oplo-h., *puls.*, sars.

Rheumatic Disorders

Extremities: Looseness, Cracking and Stiffness.

- LOOSENESS; sensation of; joints: ankles (2): aq-wild., arg.
- LOOSENESS; sensation of; joints: knees (3): aq-wild., phos., tax.
- LOOSENESS; sensation of; joints (23): aq-wild., aquilr-a., arg., **Bov.**, calen., calop-s., **Chel.**, clad-r., **Croc.**, falco-p., harp., **Med.**, **Mez.**, nat-c., **Ph-ac.**, phos., posit., **Psor.**, **STRAM.**, sumb., **Tax.**, **Thuj.**, **Visc.**

- CRACKING; joints; knees; rising, on (1): aq-wild.
- CRACKING; joints; knees; right (5): alch-v., aq-wild., *benz-ac.*, caul., mez.

- STIFFNESS; lower limbs; waking, on (6): alum., aq-wild., carb-v., cupr., meteo-a., prednisolone.
- STIFFNESS; waking, on (18): aq-sanic., aq-wild., alum., am-c., arge-p., **Ars.**, bamb-a., bos-s., crot-c., cupr., **Ferr.**, **Lach.**, **Led.**, meteo-a., ox-ac., pitu-a., posit., **Zinc.**

Extremities

- PAIN; Rheumatic; wrists; extending to; elbow (1): aq-wild.
- PAIN; Sprained, dislocated; ankles; ascending aggravates (1): aq-wild.
- PAIN; Burning, smarting; elbows; right (1): aq-wild.
- PAIN; Dislocated; ankles; ascending a height (1): aq-wild.
- PAIN; Contracting; knees (4): am-c., aq-wild., ox-ac., squil.
- PAIN; Drawing: elbows; right (6): aq-wild., **Bry.**, canth., fago., phos., sulph.

Modalities

Desire to stretch – Looseness in the joints – ankles and knees – the bones seem as if they did not fit.

Worse – Waking at night.

Worse – Lying down: throbbing, heat in occiput.

Worse – Walking: pain in sciatic nerve and looseness of knees and ankles.

Back Pain

Back

- PAIN; drawing; sponge drawn along skin, as if hot, morning on waking (1): aq-wild.
- PAIN; drawing; morning; bed, in (3): aq-wild., *hep, rhod.*
- PAIN; drawing; bed, in (6): aq-wild., ant-c., coloc., hep., rhod., valer.
- PAIN; pulsating, throbbing; cervical region; night (1): aq-wild.
- PAIN; pulsating, throbbing; cervical region (10): aq-wild., **Bamb-a., Eup-per.**, glon., lyss., manc., polyg., **Sarr.**, sulph., tarent.
- PAIN; sciatica, sciatic nerve; walking; aggravates (27).

Sensations as if:

- Brain is over-filled.
- Gnawing, sinking, empty sensation in stomach.
- Teeth seem too long.

Irritable bowel syndrome

Throat

- PAIN; oesophagus; nausea, with (2): aq-wild., xan.
- PAIN; convulsive, spasmodic; oesophagus (1): aq-wild.
- PAIN; convulsive, spasmodic (2): aq-wild., dros.
- PAIN; drawing; oesophagus (1): aq-wild.

Stomach

- APPETITE; ravenous, canine, excessive; supper, after (1): aq-wild.
- EMPTINESS, faintness; gnawing (3): aq-wild., hema-h., **Ox-ac.**
- APPETITE; gnawing (23): abies-c., abrot., adon., aq-wild., **Arg.**, arn., bacch-a., bell., **Chim-m.**, chin., coca, colch., **Fl-ac.**, iod., kreos., *lach.*, med., plac., sabad., seneg., sep., sil., ther.

Abdomen

- PAIN; menses; instead of (2): aq-wild., **Spong.**
- PAIN; cramping, gripping; menses; suppressed, from (5): aq-wild., cocc., cupr., **Mill., Puls.**

- PAIN; forenoon; eleven am.; aggravates (10): aq-wild., cast., corn., crot-h., epip., fago., mag-c., mit., tax., trom.

Rectum

- PAIN; convulsive, spasmodic; perineum (1): aq-wild.
- PAIN; convulsive, spasmodic (15): aq-wild., carbn-s., chel., colch., galph., kreos., **Lach.**, lyc., med., meteo-a., op., plb., psor., sang., **Sin-a.**

Stool

- WATERY; forenoon (3): aphis., aq-wild., sec.
- WATERY; forenoon; eleven am. (2): aq-wild., sec.
- YELLOW; gray (4): aq-wild., **Cist.**, pic-ac., sin-a.
- LIQUID, thin; dark (12).
- KNOTTY, nodular, lumpy; mucous, covered with (14).

Skin Eruptions

Back

- TINGLING, prickling; urticaria, before (1): aq-wild.

Extremities

- ERUPTIONS; vesicles; itching; fingers; second, index (2): aq-wil., pyrus-c.
- ERUPTIONS; vesicles; itching; fingers (13): ap-g., aq-wild., graph., ignis, lach., nit-ac., pyrus-c., **Ran-b.**, sabad., sal-ac., sars., sil., term-c.
- ITCHING; fingers: first, thumbs; right (1): aq-wild., second, index; left (1): aq-wild.; fourth, ring; left (2): aq-wild., *rhod.*
- ITCHING; buttocks, nates; right (2): aq-wild., mur-ac.
- ITCHING; legs; calves; left (3): aq-wild., colch., mang-acet.

Useful and/or Unusual Rubrics

Eyes

- ITCHING; Canthi; outer; right; evening (1): aq-wild.
- PAIN; Sore, bruised; canthi; inner; rubbing, on (1): aq-wild.
- PAIN; Canthi; inner; rubbing; aggravates (4): aq-wild., **Puls.**, ruta, sep.
- PAIN; Stitching; eyebrows (2): aq-wild., *petr.*
- PAIN; Tearing; eyebrows; extending to forehead (1): aq-wild.

Ears

- PAIN; pressing; meatus, external; left (2): aq-wild., bell.
- PAIN; pressing; meatus, external (7): aq-wild., *asar.*, bell., *bism.*, *nux-v.*, rheum, verat.
- PAIN; stitching; deep seated; left (3): aq-wild., aur-m-n., sarr.

Nose

- EPISTAXIS, haemorrhage; right; morning (2): aq-wild., galph.
- PAIN; burning, smarting; wings; right (6): aesc., alum., aq-wild., aur., merl., sulph.

Face

- PAIN; burning, smarting; mouth; corners; right (7): aq-wild., cymbo-ci., dros., kreos., mez., nat-c., zinc.
- PAIN; tearing; eyebrows; right (2): aq-wild., *kali-c.*
- PAIN; stitching; eyes; below (10).
- PAIN; rheumatic (45).

Mouth

- SALIVATION; bloody; talking in open air aggravates (1): aq-wild.

Urine

- SEDIMENT; crystals (14).

Male

- ERECTIONS; painful; waking, on (2): aq-wild., thuj.
- PAIN; spermatic cords; emissions, pollutions, after seminal (2): aq-wild., **Nat-p.**

Female

- MENSES; absent, amenorrhea; girls, young (22).

Chest

- CRACKING noise; sternum (7): am-c., aq-wild., *calc-p.*, *irid.*, *nat-m.*, *sulph.*, toxop-p.
- PAIN; sternum; costal cartilages; right (6): aq-wild., graph., kali-c., lina., nat-p., sulph.
- HARDNESS; lymphatic tissue, axillary (26).

Extremities

- HANGNAILS; fingernails; third, middle finger (4): aq-wild., lyc., m-aust., wye.
- HANGNAILS; fingernails (18).
- SHIVERING, shuddering; upper arms (5): aq-wild., chin., mez., pimp., teg-a.

Fever, heat

- DRY heat; pricking as from needles (5): aq-wild., bol., chin., gels., nit-ac.

Perspiration

- WAKING; on or after; dreaming, after (7): am-c., anac., aq-wild., graph., meteo-a., neod., terb-o.

Compare Related Remedies
Related level = Clinical Rubric Clusters

Remedies: Lactic acid, Oxalic acid, Picric acid, Phosphoric acid, Salicylic acid, Nitric acid.

Clinical

- DIABETES; mellitus; rheumatic (3): aq-wild., **Lac-ac.**, nat-l.

Abdomen

- EMPTINESS, faintness; gnawing (3): aq-wild., hema-h., **Ox-ac.**

Male

- ERECTIONS; easy, too (14): aq-wild., **Con.**, ferr., ferr-i., kali-c., lyc., nux-v., **Phos.**, **Pic-ac.**, **Plat.**, rhod., sabin., sumb., **Trib.**
- PAIN; emissions, pollutions, seminal; after (12): amyg-p., aq-wild., caps., cere-s., clem., dig., lyss., mag-m., **Nat-p.**, ox-ac., **Ph-ac.**, **Sal-ac.**

Head

- TENSION; scalp, external; forehead (4): anag., aq-wild., lycpr., *nit-ac.*

References

1 Van Zandvoot, R. *Complete Repertory*. Leidschendam, NL: Institute for Research in Homeopathic Information and Symptomatology, 1996. (Accessed via MacRepertory version 8.0.)
2 Eberle, H., Ritzer, F. Arzneimittelehr. Heilung von Krankheiten. In *Modernen Lebenssituationen*. Munich: Verlag Müller und Steinicke, 1999.
3 Bodich H. *The Wilhelm's Quelle: one of the most renowned springs of natural effervescent mineral water, situated at Kronthal, near Frankfort-on-the-Maine, Germany: geographical position and history of the spring, its analysis, therapeutic effects, mode of obtaining and bottling the water, and its supply to the public.* New York: S. & J. Froman, 1880. Available online at US National Library of Medicine website: http://resource.nlm.nih.gov/101229609 (Accesssed September 10th 2021.)
4 Lee A. *Homeopathic Mind Maps Vol 2. Mineral Kingdom*. Auckland: Moozoonsil Publishing, 2010. pp. 87–111.
5 Scholten J. *Homeopathy and the Elements*. Utrecht: Stichting Alonissos. pp. 309–316, 400.
6 Reference to proving by KallenbachH. In: Clarke, J.H. *Dictionary of Practical Materia Medica Vol 2 (3rd edn)*. Sittingborne, Kent: Homeopathic Book Service, 1991.

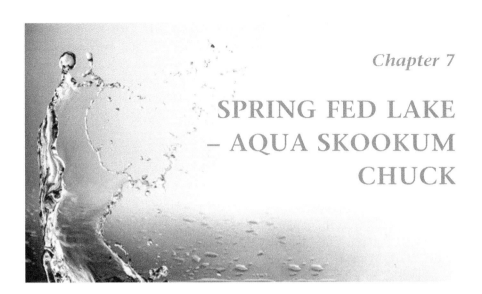

Chapter 7

SPRING FED LAKE – AQUA SKOOKUM CHUCK

AQUA SKOOKUM CHUCK

Source

The two enormous springs of Skookum Chuck arise within and form Medical Lake near Spokane Washington State USA. The town of 3070 people has the same name. The water is of a deep amber colour and almost red in the sunlight.

History

The springs were known to be medicinal by the Native Americans as far back as their oral traditions and tribal history extends and has always been held in reverence by them with free and safe access given to anyone from any tribe.

Thus spoke Quetahlguin in 1869 – last of the elders to live his whole life free:

"We have talked with the Great Spirit, and we have slept with his words in our ears. The Great Spirit is our father, and the earth is our Mother. We have a good

home and it was made for us by the Great Spirit; it is a part of us; it is our mother. In the Skookum Chuck we have a remedy for all our ailments. We have only to bathe in and drink its water and we are made well. If we sign the treaty, we will forever offend the Great Spirit; we will sign away our mother and she will cry. Her tears will dry up these lakes and we will be hungry and sick. We will go to the Skookum Chuck only to find that its waters have disappeared."[1]

Content

The following is an analysis of the salts obtained by evaporation of the water, the proportion being in grains per U. S. gallon (231 cubic inches).

- Row 2: Lithium carbonate – a trace.
- Row 3: Sodium chloride 16.370, potassium chloride 9.241, sodium carbonate 63.543, magnesium carbonate 233, aluminium oxide 175, sodium silicate 10.638, sodium bi-borate – a trace.
- Row 4: Ferrous carbonate 526, calcium carbonate 186, potassium sulphate – a trace.

Proving

There is no proving recorded in the literature; symptoms from drinking the water, from bathing and from cured cases.

Rubrics

Clinical indications

Eczema most severe on palms and/or soles: moist, painful, itchy, cracking and excoriating.
Atopic eczema and hay fever and food allergy.
Eczema begins after immunisations and NWS immunisations.
Like Sulphur eczema – skin hot red/pink, dry and cracking, must scratch, scratch until bleeds, eczema painful, but not a big aggravation from bathing.
Like routine and averse and aggravation from change especially big life changes.
The Kingdoms approach leads to a mineral, but symptoms seem similar to more than one remedy and themes/keywords from Row 2 and Row 3.

Compare/Related remedies

Related Level = Clinical Rubric Clusters

Aqua Sanicula – perforating otitis media with offensive discharge. In Aqua Sanicula the odour is of rotting fish or cheese, in Aqua Skookum Chuck the odour is of rotting meat.

Anagallis arvensis – vesicular eruptions of palms and soles which occur, heal and repeat on the same sites – see Case Report after the Aqua Skookum Chuck Case.

Carbons: Graphites, Carbo animalis, Petroleum, Kreosotum – eczema. Sulphur and Natrum sulphuricum – eczema.

Energy: Sol, Ignis, Magnetus polus arcticus, X ray.

Sarcodes and milks: Pituitary anterior, Cortisone, Lac Caninum.

Lanthanides: Neodymium carbonicum, Samarium silicatum, Yterrbium phosphoricum, Erbium sulphuricum, Dysprosium nitricum.

Acids: Nitric acid and Sulphuric acid.

Nosodes: Psorinum, Medorrhinum, Carcinosin, Variolinum, Leprominium, Malandrinum and Bacillinum.

Bowel Nosodes: Morgan Pure and Sycotic Co. (Paterson) and Dysentery Co. (Bach).

Sensitivity and vulnerability: emotional and cognitive – loss of resilience – overwhelm

- FEAR; change, of (2): *aq-skook.*, med.
- CHANGE; aversion to (12): **Aloe**, *aq-skook.*, caps., **Carb-an.**, cupr., **Kali-c.**, med., medus., podo., polyg., pot-a., sep.

- FEAR; weather, of change of (1): aq-skook.
- FEAR; wind, storm, of (17): aloe, *aq-skook.*, ars., bar-m., **Cham.**, dys-co., erech., harp., helod-c., **Lac-c.**, mang., neod-c., **Rhod.**, sama-sil., **Sep.**, thuj., ytte-p.

- MANNISH habits of; girls (12): aq-skook., carb-v., *cimic.*, cortiso., fl-ac., merc., **Nat-m.**, nux-v., petr., plat., sep., syph.

Clinical Rubric Clusters

Eruptions – palms and soles – moist, excoriating and cracking

Skin

- ERUPTIONS; eczema; vaccination, after (7): **Ammc.**, **Aq-Skook.**, **Kali-m.**, maland., **Mez.**, **Sil.**, **Thuj.**

Extremities; ERUPTIONS; eczema:

- Feet; soles (1): **Aq-Skook.**

- Hands; palms (11): anag., aq-mar., *aq-skook.*, asim., morg., prim-v., rad-br., **Ran-b.**, **Sulph.**, thul-o., **Vario.**
- Moist; hands; palms (2): aq-skook., asim.
- Sore, as if excoriated (1): **Aq-Skook.**

ERUPTIONS; excoriating, raw:

- Hands; palms (3): aq-skook., **Nat-s.**, pitu-a.
- Hands (6): aq-skook., **Nat-s.**, **Petr.**, pitu-a., sol, **Sulph.**
- CRACKS, fissures; painful; feet (3): aq-skook., carc., dys-co.
- CRACKS, fissures; feet; soles (9): acan-pl., anac-oc., **Aq-Skook.**, arist-cl., ars., *bac.*, *lepro.*, maland., merc-c.
- ERUPTIONS; crusts, scabs; feet; soles (1): aq-skook.
- ERUPTIONS; crusts, scabs; feet (7): aq-skook., bov., **Calc.**, kali-bi., mez., rhus-v., **Sil.**
- ERUPTIONS; desquamating; feet; soles (10): **Aq-Skook.**, *ars.*, chin-s., elaps, **Manc.**, parth., psil., rhus-t., sulph., thuj.
- EXCORIATION; feet; soles (11): **Aq-Sanic.**, **Aq-Skook.**, **Bar-c.**, **Calc.**, **Graph.**, **NIT-AC.**, nux-v., petr., sabad., sep., **SIL.**
- ERUPTIONS; red; fingers (3): aq-skook., graph., ignis.
- ERUPTIONS; scaly; fingers (5): aq-skook., ignis, lyc., sep., sulph.
- ERUPTIONS; excoriating, raw; hands (6): aq-skook., **Nat-s.**, **Petr.**, pitu-a., sol, **Sulph.**
- INFLAMMATION; hands; palms (4): aq-skook., bry., m-arct., pitu-a.

Skin

- ERUPTIONS; urticaria, nettle-rash; recurring (3): aq-skook., **Hep.**, stroph.
- ERUPTIONS; eczema; syphilitic (8): aq-skook., **Ars.**, **Graph.**, kreos., merc., petr., phyt., **Sars.**

Otitis Media – Perforation Tympanic Membrane and stinking discharge

Ears – DISCHARGES:

- Offensive; putrid meat, like (5): **Aq-Skook.**, **Ars.**, **KALI-P.**, **PSOR.**, **Thuj.**
- Offensive; spoiled, decayed (13): aq-sanic., **Aq-Skook.**, **Ars.**, **Bar-m.**, **Graph.**, **Hep.**, **KALI-P.**, **Lach.**, naja, pras., **PSOR.**, **TELL.**, **Thuj.**
- Ichorous (15): **Am-c.**, aq-skook., **ARS.**, **CALC.**, calc-p., **Carb-an.**, **Carb-v.**, kali-p., lach., **LYC.**, **Nit-ac.**, **PSOR.**, Sep., **Sil.**, **Tell.**

Useful or Unusual Rubrics

Generalities

- FOOD and drinks; ginger; desires (7): aq-skook., clad-r., herin., latex, meteo-a., tela, toxop-p.

Nose

- HAY fever, annual coryza; eczema, with (1): aq-skook.

Eyes

- STIES; rheumatism, after attack of (1): **Aq-Skook.**
- STIES; recurrent (17): alum., apis, aq-skook., calc-f., carbn-s., carc., **Con.**, **Graph.**, kola., lyc., med., **Psor.**, **Puls.**, **Sil.**, **Staph.**, SULPH., tub.

Chest

- TUMOURS; mammae; left (11): aq-skook., aster., brom., calc-f., calc-p., chim., con., iod., lach., phyt., psor.

Head

- ERUPTIONS; eczema; scaly (4): aq-skook., berb-a., cand-p., puls.
- ERUPTIONS; eczema; itching (7): aq-skook., cand-p., carc., gink., **Mag-c.**, plut-n., **Staph.**

Skin

- ERUPTIONS; vaccination, after (21): **Ammc.**, **Aq-Skook.**, bac., **Crot-h.**, cupre-l., dpt, **Kali-m.**, *maland.*, med., **Mez.**, nit-ac., psor., sabin., **Sars.**, sep., **Sil.**, sulph., syc-co., syph., **Thuj.**, vario.

CASE 7.1 Atopic Eczema and Grief

Context

This case illustrates: differentiation between an aggravation which heralds amelioration and a patient getting worse because the remedy is wrong.

A 70-year-old lady with grey-blonde hair and big teeth, wearing a bright blue top and cardigan and a flowery skirt presents with a severe generalised flare up of lifelong atopic eczema following the death of her husband to whom she'd been married for 44 years. Key management decisions were to decide whether the worsening after treatment with Sulphur LM1 drops would be followed by healing:

- If the doses of Sulphur were suspended for 1–2 weeks.
- If the size of dose of Sulphur LM1 were reduced to 1 drop diluted to glass 3 every third day.
- If the potency were changed.

Plus how to recognize that Sulphur is the wrong remedy and is simply making the eczema worse and how to find a more appropriate remedy for the patient.

Keywords. Atopic eczema, grief, homeopathy: Morgan Pure, Sulphur, Aqua Skookum Chuck.

Consultation June 2014

I've had eczema since I was 10 months old and its continued most of my life, some years worse than others but never gone. I was much better for a few years while taking Epogam (evening primrose oil plus Vitamin E) but gradually got dry and red and itchy again.

My husband died on New Year's Eve 2013 and my skin has been getting steadily worse since. He became ill in 2011 with a rare cancer.

Observation: tears in her eyes but she doesn't let herself cry. He had chemotherapy and surgery and radiotherapy but nothing helped. At the same time my mother got ill and went downhill rapidly. She's in a care home now half an hour away. My husband spent all of 2013 dying.

My eczema has got steadily worse with all this – it's all over me now and bad except on my face. I've seen a dermatologist and had steroid injections and tried the strong steroid creams again but even Betnovate doesn't really help – 1% Hydrocortisone seems better. I still use Betnovate diluted 1 in 4 with emollient on my wrists and hands and feet. My skin is so dry and it cracks even with lots of emollients and my eyes are so dry. I've seen an eye specialist privately and he's prescribed lubricating teardrops to use every hour and they help a bit.

I like routine. I've a big house and a huge garden. I get up and shower and put the creams on all over and have breakfast and 2 hours seem to have gone by, but I just get on even though I'm so tired.

I itch more when I sweat and when the weather is cold and dry and when the central heating is on. I'm OK abroad if it's hot. I don't seem to sweat to cool off but my feet are always sweaty and I sweat on the back of my head, my neck and hands but when I'm hot my body seems to stop sweating.

The itch can be terrible and then I must scratch and then it burns. Then my skin gets so very dry and it cracks – mainly on my hands and behind my ears and when it's bad I scratch till the skin bleeds. It is worse from 8 or 9 p.m. and worse when I sit still. 30 years ago I had some homeopathic treatment with Sulphur and it helped a lot.

We were married almost 44 years. Yes, I've cried such a lot. I prefer to cry alone. My husband was an army colonel and we made lots of good military friends and 1 couple live close and they are supportive. We were based in Germany and my husband was away a lot – fighting or training or on courses so I worked as a teacher in the military school so I was OK alone. I was working – there was the regiment and the other teachers – so my life was keeping the ship afloat. I enjoyed all the entertaining we had to do and I felt appreciated. I've had an interesting full life.

My father was a mine surveyor and my mother a housewife and we lived in the mining heartland of Yorkshire. As a child I remember being ill with my skin and with jaundice 3 or 4 times. I loved to learn and was desperate to learn to read and there was music on the radio. My father had a motorbike and sidecar and off we would all go – me and my older brother. When I started school my skin was bad and no one wanted to hold my hand. At school I was bright and artistic. I've been sewing since I was a child – I make all my own clothes and I made clothes for my husband and parents. When I started at high school I was a bit of an outsider from the village and was bullied a bit. My eczema was bad again so there were lots of rude remarks, but I developed a thick skin and to hell with you all. I passed 2 scholarships and went to Nottingham art school and studied textiles and lace. I wanted a job with regular money so went to teachers training college and became a teacher. I was invited into my first job and loved teaching. My father taught me to drive and he bought me an Austin 7 with blue leather seats.

I was very aware of security while teaching and driving – I felt very aware of danger – but I felt safe in Germany. I was always a careful driver and I learned how to change a wheel and how to maintain my car.

My husband's father was Brigadier in the army and his mother a teacher. They both died when he was 14 so he and his sister joined the army. We had no children – the decision was left to me – I've no regrets. My father died at 87 from prostate cancer and my mother is still alive at 94. My brother smokes and has COPD and asthma. There's eczema on both my parents sides.

My skin is very sensitive – to pressure and to fabrics – worse from wool and synthetics and better wearing silk, cotton and viscose. My house is very well insulated and takes little energy to heat and holds the heat well so I don't have the heating on long – I get too hot and I switch the heating off after I've had my shower in the morning but I dislike being cold. I'm comfy at 22–23 degrees at home. I usually find a coal fire too hot – even as a child it was too hot. My periods began when I was 11 and stopped when I was 51. I had a bit of flooding in my late 40s – I used to cycle to work and on the 2nd day would often have to cycle home half way to change from flooding. The Epogam stopped the hot flushes. I've never had PMT. I will argue my case but I don't shout and ball. I remember my parents shouting and it was upsetting. As a teenager I kept my thoughts to myself. I don't complain – I just get on – with my old mother and the other military wives.

My skin gets worse from eating tomato and oranges and I wear gloves to peel onions potatoes and carrots. I get anaphylactic shock from sunflower seeds but am OK with the oil. Bananas and cheese make me swell up with lots of wind but I'm OK with goat's cheese. Food isn't really a big issue for me. I love drinks – tea, water and fruit juices, tonic water, red wine and lager. I'm always very thirsty and I drink a lot. For breakfast I have half a pint of tea then porridge with lots of milk, then half a pint of tea, then half a pint of water, then half a pint of tea.

Photography was a passion for me and my husband. We catalogued our lives with photos. Mother never really bothered about learning. She liked lots of attention – she would deliberately phone when she knew I would be busy preparing for entertaining. She took a delight in disrupting my life. She spoke to me and my brother in different tones of voice – my brother could do no wrong. My father loved reading and travelling – I'm like my father in looks and build and nature.

I've only needed antibiotics a few times for dental abscesses but needed long courses. Also, for my skin a few times when the cracks get infected and ooze pus. I've an allergy to grass pollens – from June I'm sneezing and have itchy eyes. I wear *Reactolite* lenses because I'm worse in bright light. My energy is 50–60/100.

On examination: whole skin warm and pink, lots of eczema patches all over trunk and all 4 limbs, lots of little cracks wrists and hands, blood tracks from scratching all over in various stages of healing = severe atopic eczema all over except face but has eczema and bleeding cracks behind her ears.

Analysis

Is the kingdom clear?
Is the miasm clear?
What needs to be treated – eczema and grief or just eczema?
Is there a clear pattern of symptoms?
Does she need a bowel nosode now or later?

Management

Morgan Pure 30C suck 1 pill daily for 3 days and 2 weeks later begin.
Sulphur LM1 in 10% alcohol, 10 succussions before 2 drops daily in water.
Increase omega 3 oils from 2 to 3 grams a day.
Continue steroid creams and emollients.

Consultation July 2014

With the Morgan pills I had easier bowel motions and there was a subtle change in my skin – it felt and got smoother after a few days. My gut gurgled for a full 2 weeks then settled and the bowels remain easy. With Sulphur the full glass was OK but as I decreased the amount of water each day I got itchy then my skin flared up and got very itchy all over. I was a bit better on 1 drop in a big glass of water only taking a mouthful but overall my skin has been much more itchy. It has been very hot and I usually itch more when it is but I've also been tired out by the heat. My skin is improving very gradually but is still cracking and bleeding.

I'm a bit more relaxed in myself. It's become clear to me that my garden is much too big for me and the house is too big so I'm going to move. I'm sweating well in this very hot weather so that is more normal. I now feel warm on the inside and cool on the outside – so my skin is cooler. I've been having a bath in Dead Sea salt once a week and that seems to soothe my skin – for a while anyway.

On examination: her skin looks just the same to me. Some clear change from Morgan Pure and an aggravation from Sulphur glass 1– to decrease size of dose and frequency of Sulphur to 1 drop glass 3 every 3rd day. Six weeks later her skin is not settling and the aggravation from Sulphur continues even with glass 3 – it does wax and wane a bit but overall she is still worse than before treatment began.

Analysis

Aggravation from glass 3 and no big aggravation from bathing = she needs a new medicine and not Sulphur.

Atopic eczema.

Worse big changes in life: to school 1 and 2 and death of husband.

Grief processing normally apart from eczema.

Miasm clear = psora.

Good vitality: resists suppression even after a lot of steroids, no other illness and no drugs.

Unusual case = unusual remedy.

New remedy: Aqua Skookum Chuck 6x 30ml drops, 1 drop glass 3 daily till a clear change then try alternate days for 2 weeks and then every 3rd day for 2 weeks.

Consultation 23rd October 2014

There was some improvement from taking the drops daily for a week so I tried alternate days for 2 weeks and that was even better and then I tried every 3rd day for 3 doses and that wasn't so good so I've stayed on alternate days. My skin is healing and is less dry and my eyes are much less dry and I'm using the eye drops much less often.

I've begun clearing my husband's study and thrown some of my mother's old files out. I'm going to sell my house in spring because the house and garden are far too big and I'm having a new house built with a smaller garden closer to my friends and main roads and get a new life because my parents are both long lived.

My energy is better – 65–80/10 and I'm sleeping well every night. My right hip is a bit sore again and around my lower back but I have been doing a lot about the house.

On examination: almost full range of movement of right hip with a little pain at end of internal rotation; skin is better – less dry and less hot and pink – no rash or cracks behind ears – some healing on trunk and shoulders.

Management

Continue Aqua Skookum Chuck 6x 1 drop to glass 3 alternate days.
Rooibos tea for cartilage (contains manganese which is essential for
    cartilage repair).
Consider remedial massage.

Consultation 21st January 2015

My skin is improving a lot – all the horrid dryness and soreness of
the skin is gone from my whole body and down my arms and thighs.
The eczema is still there on my lower back and on my hands and from
my knees down to my feet. *Observation: still scratching wrists as she
speaks.*

I've had an X-ray which confirms osteoarthritis of my right hip but
it's not too bad and will be ages before I might need a hip replace-
ment. I can still walk for miles and I'm pain free now even standing
for hours – in fact I've only recently started sitting down to have
breakfast. I'm definitely moving house. I'm having a new house built
and hoping the move will go well. I'm making my own bread now
with a variety of flours of different grains.

In past winters my skin has been horrendous but not this year – it
used to get very, very, very dry and wrinkled very quickly but it's not
happened this year.

*On examination: normal look and feel to skin on arms and trunk and
upper limbs down to wrists and both thighs – wrists and hands and feet
still dry and red and active eczema.*

Management

Continue Aqua Skookum Chuck 6x 1 drop to glass 3 alternate days.

CASE 7.2 Anagallis arvensis

Context

Lilian is a 24-year-old woman. She has an open manner and gives her story in a simple and straightforward way.

Consultation April 1995

I have had this terrible rash on my hands for 6 months and it is just getting worse all the time. None of the creams do any good. Well I am using Dermovate 4 times a day and it only helps the itch and soreness for a while and then it all comes back. I've had 3 course of Prednisolone and it gets better while I am taking it, but it all comes back again even worse afterwards.

It started as a collection of little water blisters on both hands (shows right palm) here on both sides. The blisters soon burst and were red underneath, then they cracked and oozed and went all yellow and sore – that lasts for a few days then they heal and then it all starts again. Yes, it all starts again in the same place, and at the same time I get another group of them close to the first. Yes, they go through the same thing, they burst and the skin cracks and oozes and then they heal up. Yes, and then they all start again in the same places. It has happened like this since it all started. But more and more of my hands are getting it. It is a bit on my feet – on the bottom of my feet, but not as bad as my hands. No, nowhere else.

It just started. I had some eczema from when I was little, but it wasn't bad. It was just a few itchy patches like normal eczema. I put some cream on sometimes, but it wasn't a problem.

I got a lot of sore throats and tonsillitis in my teens, and I had a bit of acne, but it wasn't much. My periods are OK, just a bit sore the first day.

Analysis

The most striking and unusual symptom is the repetition of the eruption – new vesicles appearing on exactly the same site after initial healing. The prescription was based on recognition of this single unique keynote: that of vesicular eruptions healing and repeating on exactly the same site. This is described by Kent in his Materia Medica of Homeopathic Remedies pp 481–482 in his differentiation between the eruptions of Croton tiglium and other medicines. The rubric

Extremities; ERUPTIONS; vesicles; upper limbs; hands; healing, new vesicles appear after (1) appears in: Van Zandvoort's complete repertory, in Kent's Repertory and in Synthesis, with Anagallis arvensis as the only remedy. The repertorisation below is retrospective for illustration.

Rubrics (Complete Repertory 2005 Van Zandvoort)[2]

- Extremities; ERUPTIONS; vesicles; upper limbs; hands; healing, new vesicles appear after (1): anag.
- Extremities; ERUPTIONS; vesicles; upper limbs; hands; crops, in (1): anag.
- Extremities; ERUPTIONS; vesicles; upper limbs; hands; palms (21).
- Extremities; ERUPTIONS; vesicles; lower limbs; feet (40).

The reperotisation matrix generated by MacRepertory is shown in Figure 7.1.

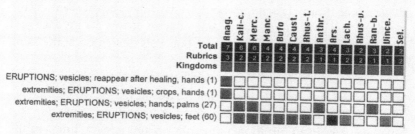

Figure 7.1 Matrix generated by MacRepertory using Complete Repertory 2015 Van Zandvoort.[1]

Management

Prescribed Anagallis arvensis 30CH one dose dry and 30ml drops to keep and use if required and advised to continue using Dermovate cream as before but to reduce use if she begins to improve.

Consultation June 1995

It's all gone away, it's amazing. Well you know you said it might get worse for a while before it started to get better, well it got really terrible. I took the remedy once and the next day it started to get really bad in my hands. It was terrible for 2 weeks the skin was all oozing and cracked and sore and the itch was nasty. The whole skin then peeled off my palms – it left a clean pink skin underneath and no blisters since. It was bad for 2 weeks then it started to heal. It has been fine for 3 or 4 weeks

During all this I got a red patch on my face. It just suddenly appeared. It was hot and bright red and spread fast from here (right temple) to across my cheek. I was a bit hot and groggy with it. I went to my GP and got penicillin for it and it just went away in a few days (*from her description the diagnosis seems to be erysipelas – consistent with the rapid resolution with penicillin*).

When my hands were starting to settle my feet got terrible. It started about 2 weeks after my hands. It was the same only worse. I couldn't walk for the pain in my feet. I had to crawl to the toilet for a few days. I was off work for a month. Then they went the same as my hands: the skin all peeled off to leave pink skin underneath, and then the skin just became normal.

When my feet were starting to get better I came out in my old eczema. It was worse than before. There were little patches of eczema all over, but it only lasted for about 10 days then it just went away.

Then, as it was fading I came out in acne. It was on my face and back like when I had it as a teenager, but it all cleared up at the same time and it hasn't come back.

My skin is completely fine. I didn't have any period pains. No, I haven't used any creams since I first saw you.

Advised to not take any further doses of Anagallis arvensis for skin unless vesicles recur but to take the drops if gets a fever illness in the next few months and see if it helps and phone me.

Telephone Consultation February 1996

I got a real dose of influenza last month, so I started taking the remedy drops like you said while I was ill with the fever and it was fine. It seemed to help quicker and better than the usual aspirin or whatever. I was still ill, but it was all over quicker. It only lasted 3 days then I was back at work and OK.

References

1 Gentry WD. Appeared in *U.S. Medical Investigator*, 1889. (Page numbers lost.)
2 Van Zandvoot, R. *Complete Repertory*. Leidschendam NL: Institute for Research in Homeopathic Information and Symptomatology, 1994. (Accessed via MacRepertory version 8.0.)

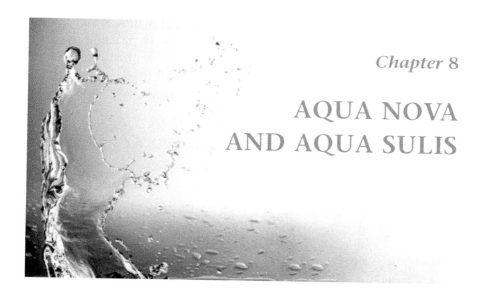

Chapter 8

AQUA NOVA
AND AQUA SULIS

AQUA NOVA

Source

Water newly created from Hydrogen & Oxygen.

Proving

The remedy was prepared by electrolysing water to Oxygen and Hydrogen gases which are then ignited to produce liquid water that may be collected.[1]

The Proving was then carried out by Misha Norland & Peter Fraser in 2009. The analysis of the provers' diaries and the transcripts of their monthly meetings took 3 years to complete. They stated,

"We cannot be absolutely sure that the distillation process removes all memory from the water and to be sure it was decided to use water that had been newly created from hydrogen and oxygen."[1]

A current of 12 volts & 20 amps DC was passed through electrodes into an electrolytic cell containing distilled water & sodium hydroxide to produce oxygen & hydrogen gases – some of the molecules of hydrogen and oxygen are monatomic and extremely vigorous. In an explosive reaction triggered by sparking the electrodes the gases unite with great exothermic vigour to produce water.

The intention, from the beginning of the proving was to use water without memory – blank.

Rubrics

Sensation as if unformed – before impressions gained from experience

- Absence of emotions – blank – featureless – empty indifference.
- Complete absence of joy – joyless.
- Static – grey – observing.
- As if there is nothing in life that could give me pleasure.

The water in Aqua Nova has experienced:

- Flow from one glass vessel to another, to another . . .
- Bubbles – during its formation – during succession at each potency step the water embraces and then releases a stream of bubbles.
- Electrical sparking.
- Being absorbed by sucrose pills.
- Being absorbed into a number of human beings who gave consent to it to affect them.

The water in Aqua Nova has never been: cloud, rain, snowflakes, icicle, glacier, river, ocean, spring, geyser or rainbow, not even once.

The water in Aqua Nova has never been part of: a dinosaur, a whale, a snail, a tiger, an octopus, a fish, a snake, fungus, a bacterium, a virus, a human, not even once.

Sensations as if invisible & not present

- People do not register my presence.
- I don't exist unless others are thinking of me.
- I'm not present – it is happening to someone else.
- Thin – as if I've lost the substance of me.
- Lightheaded – as if my head has dissolved above my eyes & is merging into the atmosphere.
- No form to the lower half of my body – only an expanse of air.
- Feet were not touching the ground.

Sensation as if in a bubble – separate

- Lonely – alone – sensation as if disconnected – as if in a bubble.
- Separated from the group – disconnected.
- I desire to be alone yet also to be part of the group.

Sensitive to energy of others & energy of places

- Take on others moods & sensations & characteristics.
- Impressionable – don't filter the impressions & don't integrate them.
- Sensation as if magnetized.
- Prescience & déjà vu.

Sensory overwhelm

- Overwhelmed by sensations & impressions – sounds, smells, seeing.
- Exquisite sensitivity to noise – noise is unbearable – a cacophony in my head – 2 sources of noise is completely unbearable – desire peace & quiet.
- Extremely sensitive to physical touch – I cannot stand it – I move away.
- As if others are so close that their face fills my whole field of vision – the closeness is uncomfortable but I don't move away.
- Prefer 1 to 1 contacts – aversion to strangers, groups, crowds – it's too much – there's too much coming at me.

Emotional overwhelm

- Resentment – dissatisfied & critical of others – I make sharp remarks.
- Aggressive towards husband – aggravated before menses & ameliorated by the flow.
- Feel threatened by men when out alone, especially in the dark.
- Fantasise about doing violence to aggressive men.
- Sensation as if accused in the group – any comment made is directed at me.
- Sensation as if the group are pulsating, raucous, greedy & like animals.
- Sensation as if there is something on my back – grabbing the back of my neck – it has its claws in me.
- Sensation as if a knife in the back.
- Image of stabbing myself in the stomach without sensation.

Explosions

- I keep thinking about explosions.
- Images of explosions.
- Explosions of anger – aggravated before menses & ameliorated by the flow.
- Explosions of aggression.
- Explosions of sexual energy.

Dreams

- A person shape shifting continuously.
- A thing shape shifting continuously.
- I must smear the house with sage to try to clear the energy in the house after some people left an unwanted presence.
- My body has the wrong clothes on – the top half & the bottom half don't match.

Physical symptoms

- Sinking sensation in solar plexus.
- Sensation of spinning but it's not vertigo.
- Sensations of heat & burning.
- Premenstrual irritability ameliorated by the flow.
- Joint pains – aching & joint stiffness.

Eyes and Vision

Sensation as if eyes:

- Too big for their sockets.
- Stabbed through with a skewer.
- Itchy & hot & swollen & heavy.
- Air blowing in eyes.
- Tunnel vision.

Caution: Aqua nova is a remedy that I cannot imagine ever prescribing to a patient. The primary risk stems from imprinting the empty slate, blank slate, memory blank induced in the proving. Of course, the provers did recover spontaneously – they were young and vigorous, but many of our patients are neither.

AQUA SULIS, BATH

Source

Water taken from the Roman Baths Museum pool in Bath, Somerset, England – the water has not been refreshed from the hot springs for almost 2,000 years.

History

The museum preserves the pool built by the Romans, dedicated to the goddess Sulis Minerva and lined with lead containing a mixture of water from all 3 hot springs rising at Bath – the Cross spring, King's spring and Heitling spring. At its heyday the waters flowed through the pool giving a bathing temperature of 44 degrees Celsius.

The Romans built their pool on the same site as an ancient pool held in reverence for thousands of years by the Britons and Celts – a site of worship of the Goddess. The name is likely to have arisen from the proto-German root "sule" = soul.

Content

The mineral contents of the 3 hot springs of Bath springs are very similar. The water used in this proving was cold, taken from a pool whose water has not been renewed for a very long time – the pool and sides are stained deep orange from the oxidation of ferrous to ferric salts and ferric oxide. The water has lost the radioactive gases Radon^{222} and Helium^4 yet retains Radium^{226} Uranium^{234} and Uranium^{238}.

Mineral contents: sulphates, bicarbonates, chlorides and nitrates and oxides and silicates of Calcium, Sodium, Magnesium, Potassium, Strontium, · Iron, Barium, Boron, Manganese, Radium and Uranium, with traces of Bromine and Iodine – elements and salts from rows 2–7 of the periodic table.

Proving

The Proving was carried out by Mary English and Usha Pearce.[2]

Rubrics

Sensitivity and vulnerability: emotional and cognitive – loss of resilience – overwhelm

- Calm and clear and quiet – clarity of emptiness – a sensation of equilibrium.
- Faith and strength – I feel Christ in my heart – I am responsible for the path I walk.
- Creativity – silver strands – silver threads of stories.
- I feel energized and creative.
- I feel energetic like a warrior.
- I feel bubbly.

- I feel excitable and giggly and a bit hysterical and find things amusing which are not then feel fuzzy as if I've taken mushrooms.

- I'm fed up and irritated – worse waiting in traffic, I get very bad tempered.
- I feel such violent anger – I threw a glass in the sink and smashed it and it cut my hand and felt insensibly outraged.
- I feel like fuming and shouting and screaming and end up crying from anger.
- Rage: a dark rage at the deepest part of my soul.

Desire to beget children and be a parent

- Desire to be pregnant – a deep wanting to have a baby.
- Sensation as if there is a clock ticking in my womb – it's only a matter of time and I will be pregnant.
- Sensation as if the only thing that matters is to create new life.
- Sensation as if a great emptiness inside as once again I'm not pregnant.

Children

- Dream I am sitting on a water lily with my sons.
- Dream of a wraith-like child – I think he is my son – he is white and ghostly and might die.
- Sensation as if I want/need to protect my daughter from the world.
- Sensation as if my son will be murdered by his father.

Expressions of femininity – fertility and libido

- Sensation as if energy flowing in my womb.
- Sensation as if quivering in my womb.
- Sensation of a whoosh over and in my womb.
- Sensation as if self-fertilising – and warm and damp.
- Sensation as if a river in womb.
- The truth about sex is the penis entering the womb – it is a truth about love – I want to be stirred by a man.
- Feeling sexually charged.
- Desire to have sex with many men.
- I feel a deep love for my partner – a desire to love and to be loved.
- I feel rejected by my partner and utterly devastated.
- Loss of libido – I don't even think about sex.

Water and thirst

- Desire to shower.

- Desire to bathe in deep water and with a shower on like a waterfall.
- Dreams of water: bathing, swimming, floods, dead body in the sea which sinks then rises again.
- Dream of contamination in the sea like smallpox.
- Dream I was washing my hair with shampoo and then all my hair fell out.
- Dream of a dirty toilet and the flush wasn't working and the sink wasn't working so I can't wash my hands.
- Thirsty and desire for water.
- Wakes through night thirsty.
- Dryness of mucous membranes: mouth and throat and eyes.
- Copious coryza – excoriating.

Sensations as if

- The remedy is from the depths of the earth – from its core.
- Something jagged and rough – like shards, brittle.
- An elemental energy.
- An ancient time – in England in the time of the pagans.
- Life from the beginning of time (compare Aqua Marina).
- A shining golden light in a golden landscape.
- Burning in vagina.

Physical symptoms

- Chilliness – persistent and internal and I just can't get warm.
- Hard to get to sleep because I feel so cold.
- Coldness of hands and feet worse in the evening.
- Pain in throat, worse on right side, better drinking hot tea.
- Rawness in throat worse drinking cold water.
- Abdominal bloating.
- Profuse leucorrhoea.

References

1 Norland M, Fraser P. The School of Homeopathy, Devon, 2006. Available online at: http://www.hominf.org/aquanova/aqnointr.htm (Accessed September 17th 2021.)
2 English M. *Proving Aqua Sulis*. Available online at: www.maryenglish.com (Accessed 21st June 2021.)

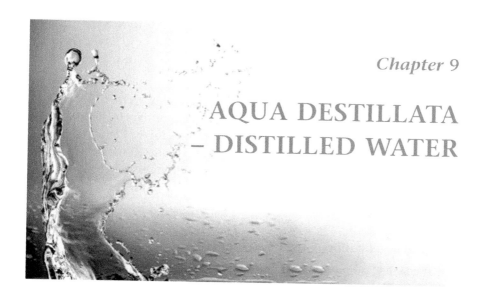

Chapter 9

AQUA DESTILLATA – DISTILLED WATER

AQUA DESTILLATA – DISTILLED WATER

Source

Distilled Water Ph. Eur. produced in Germany to European Pharmacopea standard was used – this is almost entirely pure water – purchased from a local pharmacy by Monika Kittler the proving director.

Distillation involves heating the water in a glass vessel till hot vapour/steam rises through glass piping to another glass vessel where the vapour collects and condenses and cools as liquid water. The minerals in the original source water are left behind in the first vessel.

The source of the water used by the distilling company is not known.

Proving

The proving was carried out by Monika Kittler in 2001.[1]

The first stage was a group trituration to C4:

"I decided on the classic trituration according to §270 Organon, whereby I did not, as Hahnemann prescribes, triturate up to C3, but one potency step further

up to C4, in the hope that the information of the distilled water would then be more clearly revealed. I imagined that if I believed in the possibility of this path during the trituration and, so to speak, helped shape the process with this belief and trust, the water would convey itself to me".

The second stage involved the whole proving group (6 women and 3 men) making liquid potencies 5 to 30C in the Hahnemannianian method then taking a dose of 30C daily till symptoms were produced.

My impression of the proving is that it was conducted with correctness, attention to detail and with a cheerful respect, even reverence.

Rubrics

Desire to beget children and be a parent

- PREGNANT, desire to be (3): aq-des., brachy-s-p., onc-t.
- CHILDREN; desires to; have, to beget, to nurture (8): aq-des., aq-taosc., lim-b-c., lsd, nat-m., *onc-t.*, ox-ac., *plac.*
- CHILDLESS, ailments from being (10): aq-des., aq-taosc., aur., lac-h., lim-b-c., lsd, nat-m., *onc-t.*, ox-ac., plac.

Sensitivity and vulnerability: emotional and cognitive – loss of resilience – overwhelm

- LOQUACITY; Morning (1): aq-des.
- DELUSIONS, imaginations; Floor; wobbling, is (1): aq-des.

Chest

- ANXIETY; mammae (2): aq-des., **PHOS.**

Dreams

- Ice cream (1): aq-des.
- Blood; blood vessels (2): aq-des., pyrus-c.
- Rabies, of (2): aq-des., oryc-c.
- Trees, of; chopping down (5): aq-des., cordy-a., lac-eq., stoi-k., succ.
- Fire; house, building, on (7): aq-des., bell., gink., kali-c., lac-lup., mag-s., plut-n.

Water and thirst

Dreams

- Clouds; can touch (1): aq-des.
- Clouds (3): aq-des., mus-m., phasc-c.
- Fog, of (1): aq-des.

- Water; blood, becomes (1): aq-des.
- Snow (24): *amet.*, aq-des., art-v., bapt., brass., caras., caul., cyg-b., falco-p., galeoc-c., harp., hippo-k., hydrog., **Kreos.**, lap-be-e., lim-b-c., *mand.*, meteo-a., niob., onc-t., ozone, plut-n., tax., thea.

Stomach

- THIRST; night; waking, on (20): acon., agath-a., aloe, aq-des., *aq-hoch.*, bacch-a., berb., bry., calad., carb-an., carc., cina, **Coff.**, cyg-c., kola., **Nat-s.**, **Stram.**, tax., teucr-s., vip.

Clinical Rubric Clusters

Heartburn

- Chocolate, after (1): aq-des.
- Spices, condiments, piquant, highly seasoned food, after (1): aq-des.
- Night (13): aq-des., chin., coc-c., con., conch., dysp-n., *eug.*, ferr-p., kali-bi., **Merc.**, posit., ptel., **Rob.**

- NAUSEA; spices, condiments, piquant, highly seasoned food, after (1): aq-des.
- APPETITE; increased, hunger in general; menses; before (8): agath-a., aq-des., croc., lat-h., mag-c., puls., sep., spong.

Rheumatic disorders

- Inflammatory arthritis – mainly large joints lower limbs and tendonitis.

Generalities

- PAIN Joints: burning and stitching.
- INFLAMMATION; Tendons and synovitis.

Patellar bursitis, jerking and pain in knees

Extremities

- PAIN; knees; patella; cold aggravates (1): aq-des.
- PAIN; knees; patella; behind, bursitis (7): aq-des., arg-n., arn., **RHUS-T.**, sep., slag, tama.
- PAIN; knees; patella; motion; aggravates (8): aml-n., aq-des., berb., cact., coc-c., ery-a., ph-ac., staph.
- PAIN; burning, smarting; knees; ascending stairs aggravates (2): aq-des., sulph.

- CRACKING; joints; knees; descending stairs (4): aq-des., caul., **CAUST.**, hura.

- JERKING; knees; inner, medial, night (1): aq-des.
- JERKING; lower limbs; night (5): aq-des., **Arg-n.**, kali-bi., lyc., **Phos.**

Back

- PAIN; drawing; sacral region; menses, during (4): aq-des., cham., con., zing.

Skin eruptions

Face

- ERUPTIONS; eyes; below (8): aq-des., dulc., guai., hep., plut-n., sel., tax., thuj.
- ERUPTIONS; eczema; mouth; around (17): **Ant-c.**, aq-des., aur., bac., bov., calc., erb., graph., hib, kali-sil., led., lyc., **Mez.**, mur-ac., **Nat-m.**, prim-o., **Rhus-v.**

Useful or Unusual Rubrics

Urine

- EATEN, odour of what was (1): aq-des.

Sleep

- WAKING; midnight; after; four am.; five am., until (10): aq-des., aur-m-n., aur-s., cortico., latex, nux-v., ptel., sulph., telo-s., verat.

Generalities

- FOOD and drinks; Meat; desires; must have (6): aq-des., **Calc.**, *graph.*, **Nux-v.**, **Staph.**, **Sulph.**

Related remedies – share and compare level
Aqua Destillata is in several or many rubrics with certain other remedies. This correspondence within rubrics can represent shared: sensation or theme, or modality or quality or site of pain, or general symptom like food desire or a clinical rubric cluster like heartburn.

The Share and Compare Level is quite a low level of correspondence – we are both in the same rubric – "Hello, do we know each other?"

The Clinical Rubric Cluster is a higher level because it has multiple rubrics centred round a clinical condition so is also clinically useful.

The highest level of relationship is shared Vital Sensation – fish are one of the most closely related families to the Aqua not just because fish live in water but because both remedy families share 2 Vital Sensations: Flow and Bubble.

The theme placed first for Aqua Destillata is Desire to Beget Children and Be a Parent, and in those rubrics there is also Oncorhyncus tshawytscha, sockeye salmon.

- PREGNANT, desire to be (3): aq-des., brachy-s-p., onc-t.
- CHILDREN; desires to; have, to beget, to nurture (8): aq-des., aq-taosc., lim-b-c., lsd, nat-m., *onc-t.*, ox-ac., *plac.*
- CHILDLESS, ailments from being (10): aq-des., aq-taosc., aur., lac-h., lim-b-c., lsd, nat-m., *onc-t.*, ox-ac., plac.

Two other remedies in these 3 rubrics come as no surprise: Placenta humana and Lac humanum representing nurture within the uterus and after birth.

Let's see if there are other milks and then move on to other remedy families or single remedies related to Aqua Destillata.

Milks – Share and Compare – Lac equinum, Lac lupinum and Lac caninum

- DREAMS; Trees, of; chopping down (5): aq-des., cordy-a., lac-eq., stoi-k., succ.
- DREAMS; Fire; house, building, on (7): aq-des., bell., gink., kali-c., lac-lup., mag-s., plut-n.
- Extremities; WARTS; fingers; third, middle (6): aq-des., berb., lac-c., lach., rosm., sal-ac.

Acids

Oxalic acid shares main Aqua theme: Desire to Beget Children and be a Parent plus Childless, ailments from being.

Share and Compare: Carbolic acid, Nitric acid, Phosphoric acid, Lactic acid, Salicylic acid and Fluoric acid.

Oxalic acid

- CHILDREN; desires to; have, to beget, to nurture (8): aq-des., aq-taosc., lim-b-c., lsd, nat-m., *onc-t.*, ox-ac., *plac.*
- CHILDLESS, ailments from being (10): aq-des., aq-taosc., aur., lac-h., lim-b-c., lsd, nat-m., *onc-t.*, ox-ac., plac.

Share and Compare for the other 6 acids

Extremities

- COLDNESS, chilliness; legs; bones, tibia (8): aq-des., berb., carb-ac., **Mosch.**, nit-ac., ph-ac., **Rhus-t.**, samb.
- WARTS; fingers; third, middle (6): aq-des., berb., lac-c., lach., rosm., sal-ac.

Mouth

- REDNESS; fiery; tongue (13): **APIS**, aq-des., **Ars.**, **Bell.**, calc-s., **Canth.**, **Crot-h.**, **Fl-ac.**, **Phyt.**, **Pyrog.**, **Sang.**, sulph., zinc-m.
- ERUPTIONS; eczema; mouth; around (17): **Ant-c.**, aq-des., aur., bac., bov., calc., erb., graph., hib, kali-sil., led., lyc., **Mez.**, mur-ac., **Nat-m.**, prim-o., **Rhus-v.**

Phosphorus: Related Level: Suppression of Emotions – Sublimation of libido

- Chest; ANXIETY; mammae (2): aq-des., **PHOS.**
- Extremities; JERKING; Lower limbs; night (5): aq-des., **Arg-n.**, kali-bi., lyc., **Phos.**

Energy remedies – Ultraviolet light – Share and Compare

- DREAMS; Desert, of (5): aq-des., herin., maia-l., *sil.*, uv-lux.
- DREAMS; Pork, boars (4): aq-des., merl., succ., uv-lux.
- DREAMS; light (11): *amet.*, aq-des., coff., *galeoc-c.*, kola., lach., mus-m., nept-m., perla, ratt-n., uv-lux.

Gemstones – Amethyst, Pearl and Amber – Share and Compare

- DREAMS; light (11): *amet.*, aq-des., coff., *galeoc-c.*, kola., lach., mus-m., nept-m., perla, ratt-n., uv-lux.
- DREAMS; Pork, boars (4): aq-des., merl., succ., uv-lux.

Birds – Macaw, Bald Eagle, Bewick Swan, Whooper Swan, Peregrine Falcon and Californian Roadrunner

Generalities

- FOOD and drinks; bananas; desires (19): adam., ana-i., aq-des., ara-m., cer-i., *fic-sp.*, haliae-lc., ignis, kali-c., lant-c., med., ozone, phos., puls., sep., syph., **Ther.**, **Tub.**, tung.

- DREAMS; Snow (24): *amet.*, aq-des., art-v., bapt., brass., caras., caul., cyg-b., falco-p., galeoc-c., harp., hippo-k., hydrog., **Kreos.**, lap-be-e., lim-b-c., *mand.*, meteo-a., niob., onc-t., ozone, plut-n., tax., thea.

Above see Aqua Destillata in DREAMS; Snow with: Sockeye Salmon and Goldfish and Seahorse; Amethyst and Emerald; Bewick Swan and Peregrine Falcon and Californian Roadrunner; Hydrogen and Ozone.

Reference

1 Kittler M. *Aqua Distillata – Die Prufung*. Zweibrücken D: Karl-Josef Müller, Vedriag, 2001.

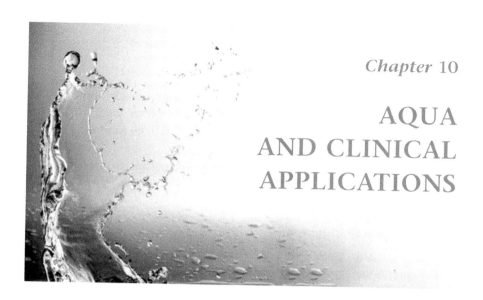

Chapter 10

AQUA
AND CLINICAL
APPLICATIONS

The beautiful paradox of case analysis exists in the tension between the totality of symptoms and the most unique, striking, strange, rare and peculiar symptoms as first described by Hahnemann in the *Organon*, Aphorisms 7 and 153.

When to consider an Aqua during case taking and case analysis

- Heuristic: Unusual case = Unusual remedy.
- Kingdom approach when the mineral kingdom is clear and yet:
- Themes and keywords of more than one row of the periodic table.
- Themes and keywords of more than two columns of the periodic table.
- Strange, Rare and Peculiar symptom and Repertory search leads to an *Aqua*.
- Key Symptom or Clinical Rubric Cluster of an *Aqua*.
- Pattern or totality recognition of a specific *Aqua*.

Clinical disorders which can present with Aqua symptom patterns

- Anxiety state.
- Headaches and migraine.

- Rheumatic disorders: osteoarthritis, inflammatory arthritis and back pain.
- Irritable Bowel Syndrome and constipation.
- Skin disorders – eczema, boils, vesicular eruptions, cracks and corns.
- Heartburn and acid reflux, hiatus hernia and peptic ulcer.
- Exhaustion – Mental and Physical – Chronic fatigue syndrome and ME.
- Heavy metal toxicity: Aqua Cross Spring Bath, Aqua Gastein, Aqua Weilbach.

Aqua containing Lithium salts

- Aqua Carlsbad, Aqua Gastein, Aqua Gettysburg, Aqua Kronthal, Aqua Sanicula, Aqua Teplitz and Aqua Wiesbaden.
- Care should be taken when prescribing one of the Aqua above to a patient with Bi-Polar Disorder taking Lithium Carbonate/Citrate as a mood stabiliser. It is most unlikely that there would be any change in the serum lithium level. Nevertheless, close attention to indicators of early hypomania is time well spent at review appointments. The symptoms/signs can be subtle: going to bed later and getting up early, spending more money, speaking more quickly and delighted with all the energy this new remedy is giving.

Aqua containing Arsenic salts

- Aqua Bondonneau, Aqua Gastein, Aqua Levico, Aqua Reinerz, Aqua Vichy Grande Grille and Aqua Wiesbaden.
- Homeopathic treatment is remarkably safe, yet arsenic is toxic, so the above Aqua should be prescribed at 12C or higher, or as Q4 or higher.
- Sensitive patients can begin to imprint remedies from repeated doses of a homeopathic remedy, e.g. as a Q/LM potency.
- Should a sensitive patient report sustained rise in anxiety with restless pacing and inability to rest until everything is in its proper place then they may be imprinting the arsenic salt in the Aqua and the remedy should be stopped.

Aqua Wiesbaden contains both Lithium and Arsenic salts.

Clinical Rubric Cluster – Anxiety state – Aqua Marina

Aqua Marina can be considered for anxiety state in the same way that you may consider Arsenicum album or Calcarea carbonica.

- ANXIETY; motion; ameliorates; fast (2): aq-mar., saroth.
- ANXIETY; afternoon; ameliorates (2): aq-mar., tab.
- ANXIETY; drinks, cold, ameliorate; ice cold (2): agar-em., aq-mar.
- ANXIETY; drinks, cold, ameliorate (4): **Acon.**, **Agar-em.**, aq-mar., sulph.
- ANXIETY; perspiration; ameliorates (4): agar., aq-mar., calc., camph.

- ANXIETY; afternoon; aggravates, two pm. – four pm. (2): aq-mar., **Coc-c.**
- FEAR; looked at, when (10): aq-mar., *ars.*, bar-c., calc., germ., med., meli., ratt-n., rhus-t., tub.

Clinical Rubric Cluster – Anxiety state and Other Aqua

- ANXIETY; coffee; aggravates (5): aq-bart., **CHAM.**, ign., **Nux-v.**, stram.
- ANXIETY; heart region; evening (7): anag., aq-carl., bell., brom., cench., hydrog., Puls.
- ANGUISH; night; waking, on (4): aq-kiss., kali-br., **Nat-s.**, **Nux-v.**

- FEAR; change, of (2): *aq-skook.*, med.
- FEAR; dentist, of going to (6): *aq-hoch.*, calc., lyc., nat-glut., puls., tub.
- FEAR; examinations, of; medical (6): ant-t., aq-sanic., nit-ac., phos., puls., tub.
- FEAR; lightning, of (9): aq-taosc., bell., cycl., dig., dpt, lach., phos., phys., sil.

- EXCITEMENT, excitable; morning; rising, on (3): *aloe*, aq-carl., iber.
- FIRE; thinks and talks of (5): acan-pl., aq-taosc., bacch-a., **Calc.**, gink.
- DREAMS; fire; house, building, on (7): aq-des., bell., gink., kali-c., lac-lup., mag-s., plut-n.
- RESTLESSNESS, nervousness; night; waking (7): agar., aq-kiss., caust., lyc., par., saroth., sep.
- RESTLESSNESS, nervousness; midnight; after; four a.m. (5): aq-wild., clem., kreos., nit-ac., trom.
- SADNESS; Fear, with; evil, of impending (5): aq-sanic., **Aur.**, calc., **Caust.**, **KALI-I.**

Clinical Rubric Cluster – Headaches and Migraine

Remedies: A. qua Sanicula, Aqua Wildbad, Aqua Hall, Aqua Carlsbad, Aqua Teplitz and Aqua Kissingen – these can be considered for headaches and migraine in the same way that you may consider Belladonna or Sanguinaria or Spigelia.

PAIN, headache:

- Wandering; spot touched with fingers, to (2): aq-sanic., asaf.

- Bursting; stool; straining at (4): alum., aq-sanic., **Ind.**, **Rat.**
- Pulsating, throbbing; waking, on (5): aq-wild., ozone, *sia-c.*, sulph., tarent.
- Stitching; occiput; extending; eye, to, right (2): aq-sanic., **Sang.**
- Stitching; occiput; right; extending to: Forehead (2): aq-sanic., chel.
- Drawing; vertex; right (2): aq-lipp., *spig.*
- Drawing; vertex; extending to; temple (3): aq-hall, bor., chel.
- Burrowing; sides (7): aq-carl., **Agar.**, bry., chin., clem., phos., rat.

- Sore, bruised; occiput; pressure; aggravates (4): aq-sanic., cimic., cupr-ar., tab.
- Sore, bruised; scalp, external; touching hair aggravates (6): **Alum.**, aq-tep., lycpr., salx-n., **Sil.**, **Spig.**
- Forehead; bending head; backward; ameliorates (5): aq-sanic., **Bell.**, **Ign.**, thuj., verat.
- Riding in a carriage; ameliorates (8): **Aq-Sanic.**, brom., graph., **Kali-n.**, merc., **Nit-ac.**, olea, stoi-k.
- Tearing; motion; ameliorates (8): *act-sp.*, *aq-carl.*, caps., kali-i., mur-ac., **Rhod.**, **Rhus-t.**, sulph.
- Occiput; heaviness, with (3): aq-mar., bapt., cic.
- Occiput; ascending stairs aggravates (8): aq-carl., **Bell.**, **Carb-v.**, ip., mosch., nat-s., pic-ac., sep.

Vision

- DIPLOPIA; headache; with (8): aq-kiss., **Gels.**, ger., kali-chl., morph-m., neod-s., phyt., stroph.
- SPARKS; headache; during (10): am-c., aq-hall, ars., **Chel.**, chin-s., lach., lyss., **MAG-P.**, phos., **Pic-ac.**

Hearing

- ROARING; headache, during (16): aq-hall, aur., bor., chen-a., **Chin.**, **Chin-s.**, chlf., ferr., gels., onos., paeon., *plat.*, sang., **Sil.**, **Staph.**, sulfon.

Clinical Rubric Cluster – Back Pain

Remedies: Aqua Sanicula, Aqua Teplitz, Aqua Wildbad, Aqua Hall and Aqua Destillata.

Clinical Rubric Cluster – Aqua Sanicula and Back Pain

Back

- PAIN; lumbar region, lumbago; lying; ameliorates; side, on (4): aq-sanic., des-ac., nat-s., zinc.

- PAIN; lumbar region, lumbago; exertion; ameliorates; gentle (2): aq-sanic., coriand.
- PAIN; lumbar region, lumbago; exertion; ameliorates (5): aq-sanic., coriand., galeoc-c., ozone, **Rad-br.**
- PAIN; exertion; ameliorates (8): aq-sanic., coriand., galeoc-c., glyc-g., ozone, **Rad-br.**, ruta, **Sep.**

- PAIN; break, as if back would; rising, on (4): aq-sanic., carb-an., chel., sul-i.
- PAIN; burning, smarting; sacral region; sitting, while (4): aq-sanic., bor., helon., kreos.
- PAIN; sprained, dislocated, as if; lumbar region; vertebra, fifth (2): aq-sanic., sarr.
- PAIN; muscles; psoas (5): all-s., aq-sanic., arg., *aur.*, crot-c.
- TENSION; short, as if muscles too (5): aq-sanic., aur., hyos., lyc., sulph.

Neck

- PAIN; stitching; sides; turning head (3): aq-sanic., coc-c., dig.

Clinical Rubric Cluster – Other Aqua and Back Pain

- PAIN; paralytic; lumbar region; evening (3): alum., aq-bart., **Kalm.**
- PAIN; lumbar region, lumbago; extending to; calves (6): aq-tep., berb., ozone, ph-ac., pitu-a., zinc.

- STIFFNESS; painful; motion aggravates (8): aq-vichy-g., cinch., *cocc.*, dros., **Guai.**, **Led.**, **Mez.**, rhus-t.

Clinical Rubric Cluster – Rheumatic disorders and Aqua Sanicula

Extremities

- PAIN; Burning, smarting; feet; soles; uncover, inclination to (7): **AQ-SANIC.**, **Cham.**, helo., **Lach.**, **Med.**, **Sang.**, **Sulph.**

- PAIN; Constant; shoulders (3): aq-sanic., ind., verat-v.
- PAIN; shoulders; motion; aggravates; arm, of; behind back (5): **Aq-Sanic.**, **FERR.**, **Ign.**, **Rhus-t.**, sep.
- PAIN; Sore, bruised; hands; left (3): aq-sanic., pitu-a., succ.
- PAIN; rheumatic; hips; left (11): **Acon.**, ant-t., **Aq-Sanic.**, ba-sv., equis., ferr., ferr-p., lyc., nat-m., sang., **Stram.**
- PAIN; sprained, dislocated; feet; left (5): *anac.*, aq-sanic., **Hyper.**, lac-cpr., *nat-m.*

- STIFFNESS; hands; waking, on (11): alum., aq-sanic., **Ars.**, bamb-a., bos-s., cupr., **Ferr.**, **Lach.**, **Led.**, pitu-a., posit.

Clinical Rubric Cluster – Other Aqua and Rheumatic Disorders

Extremities

- LOOSENESS; sensation of; joints; ankles (2): aq-wild., arg.
- COLDNESS, chilliness; painful; lower limbs (4): aq-tep., caust., chel., **Syph.**

- PAIN; sprained, dislocated; toes; right (2): aq-wild., syph.
- PAIN; broken, as if; hips; walking, on (2): aq-tep., dros.
- PAIN; toes; frozen: after being (3) and formerly frozen (3): agar., aq-carl., phos.

- PAIN; violent; shoulders; right (3): aq-tep., carb-ac., *chel.*
- PAIN; tearing; drawing; scapulae (2): aq-tep., stann.
- PAIN; elbows; bones; rest, during (4): agar., aq-hall, arg-n., aur-m-n.
- PAIN; elbows; alternating with pain in; shoulders (2): aq-tep., kalm.
- PAIN; violent; wrists (5): act-sp., apoc-a., aq-tep., **Caul.**, hipp.
- PAIN; pressing; dull; hip region (2): aq-carl., zinc.
- PAIN; knees; patella; behind, bursitis (7): aq-des., arg-n., arn., **RHUS-T.**, sep., slag, tama.

- PAIN; rheumatic; tendons (7): aq-get., arn., **Colch.**, form-ac., phyt., rhod., **Rhus-t.**
- PAIN; rheumatic; rest; ameliorates (6): aq-get., bry., caust., colch., mag-p., *squil.*

Generalities

- PAIN; burning, smarting; bones; night (7): aq-get., **Caust.**, dros., kali-bi., **Mez.**, **Ph-ac.**, phos.

Clinical Rubric Cluster – irritable bowel syndrome

Aqua Carlsbad and Irritable bowels syndrome

Stomach

- HICCOUGH; breakfast; after (4): alum., aq-carl., **Tarent.**, **Zinc.**
- PAIN; Pressing; supper, after (9): am-c., aq-carl., **Calc.**, lyc., nat-c., puls., seneg., zinc., zinc-o.

Abdomen

- HEAVINESS as from a load or weight; drinking aggravates (3): aq-carl., **Asaf.**, sin-a.
- RUMBLING noise; coffee ameliorates (3): aq-adel., aq-carl., phos.
- TENSION; dinner, after (5): aq-carl., cycl., nit-ac., plat., sulph.

- PULSATION; lying, while (5): aloe, aq-carl., aran-ix., **Coloc.**, plb.
- CONSTRICTION; bowels (8): *aq-carl.*, astac., chion., **Coloc.**, **Plb.**, **Spig.**, **Ter.**, **Thuj.**

Clinical Rubric Clusters – other Aqua and irritable bowel syndrome

Remedies: Aqua Sanicula, Aqua Vichy Grande Grille, Aqua Adelheid, Aqua Kissingen, Aqua Hall, Aqua Franzensbad and Aqua Reinerz.

Stomach

- FULLNESS; loosen clothing, must (2): aq-sanic., dys-co.
- DISTENSION; supper; after (6): aq-sanic., *cadm.*, calc., chin., *ign.*, zinc.
- DISTENSION; eating; while (10): apoc., aq-sanic., *cann-i.*, con., dulc., ferr-ma., germ., ign., nat-p., *sars.*
- PAIN; Burning; salivation, with (3): aq-vichy-g., *brom.*, ter.

Abdomen

- FULLNESS; stool; ameliorates (2): aq-rein., colch.
- GURGLING; eating; after (5): aq-sanic., bacch-a., *merc.*, tus-fa., *zinc.*
- RETRACTION; convulsive, spasmodic (9): *act-sp.*, aq-kiss., *chel.*, *plat.*, plb., plb-chr., stram., **Sul-ac.**, *tab.*

PAIN

- Cramping, gripping; umbilical region; extending; downward (3): aq-hall, ind., plat.
- Morning; stool; ameliorates (6): aq-vichy-g., ars., ferr., indg., mez., phys.
- Bed; in; ameliorates (6): aq-franz., **Ars.**, **Coloc.**, sin-n., staph., symph.
- Cramping, gripping; stool, as before (7): aphis., aq-lipp., chel., mang., raph., sin-a., **Trom.**
- Cramping, gripping; morning; rising; on (8): aq-vichy-g., digin., ham., nat-m., ruta, trif-p., *trom.*, **Zinc-val.**

Rectum

- CONSTRICTION, closure, contraction; standing; ameliorates (2): **Alum.**, aq-sanic.
- INVOLUNTARY stool; attention on sphincter, must keep (5): **Aloe**, **Apoc.**, **Aq-Sanic.**, **Gels.**, **Phos.**
- URGING, desire; eating; during (8): aloe, aq-sanic., **Ars.**, **Chin.**, dios., **Ferr.**, *sep.*, trom.

Clinical Rubric Cluster – Constipation

Remedies: Aqua Sanicula and Aqua Marina. Compare: Opium and Natrum muriaticum.

Rectum; CONSTIPATION:

- Inactivity; chronic (4): alum., aq-sanic., bac., sep.
- Seashore, at; aggravates (4): *aq-mar.*, lyc., **Mag-m.**, **Nat-m.**
- Urging; absent: Accumulation of stool, until large (8): *alum.*, **Anac.**, **Aq-Sanic.**, **Bry.**, meli., **Nat-m.**, **Op.**, **Sulph.**
- Home, when away from (16): **Alum.**, ambr., aq-mar., **Germ.**, **Ign.**, **Lyc.**, **M-arct.**, mag-acet., med., nat-m., **Nux-v.**, **Op.**, **PLAT.**, **Sep.**, sil., sile-c.
- HARD; size immense, comes out in parts (2): **Aq-Sanic.**, mez.
- HEAVY (4): **Aq-Sanic.**, bac., nat-m., salx-f.
- FORCIBLE, sudden, gushing; impacted (6): **Aq-Sanic.**, **Calc.**, **Nat-m.**, **Sel.**, **Sep.**, **Sil.**

Skin Eruptions and Ulcers

Remedies: Aqua Skookum Chuck, Aqua Sanicula, Aqua Marina and Aqua Bartfelder.

Skin

- ERUPTIONS; eczema; vaccination, after (7): **Ammc.**, **Aq-Skook.**, **Kali-m.**, maland., **Mez.**, **Sil.**, **Thuj.**

Extremities

- ERUPTIONS; eczema; hands; palms (11): anag., aq-mar., *aq-skook.*, asim., morg., prim-v., rad-br., **Ran-b.**, **Sulph.**, thul-o., **Vario.**

Skin

- ULCERS; discharging, suppurating; offensive; fish brine, like (4): aq-sanic., **Graph.**, **Lach.**, **Tell.**

Face

- ERUPTIONS; vesicles; cheeks (6): aq-mar., buni-o., electr., **Euph.**, syc-co., valer.

Extremities

- ERUPTIONS; vesicles; white; red; areola, hands (2): aq-sanic., uran-n.

- ERUPTIONS; urticaria, nettle-rash; morning (4): aq-bart., **Bell.**, bov., chin.

- ERUPTIONS; urticaria, nettle-rash; exertion aggravates (9): aq-sanic., **Ant-c.**, apis, calc., **Con.**, hep., **Nat-m.**, **Psor.**, **Urt-u.**

- ERUPTIONS; boils, furuncles; wrists (2): aq-sanic., **Iod.**
- ERUPTIONS; pustules; fingers; first, thumb (2): aq-sanic., cic.

Aqua and Cracks and Corns and Excoriation

The rubrics show useful rubrics for cracks and corns, with what readers know as major skin remedies, like Graphites, Petroleum, Sulphur and Sepia, and I want to show that right in there with the skin polycrests are Aqua.

Extremities

- ERUPTIONS; crusts, scabs; cracks, full of, hands (4): **Anthr.**, **Aq-Sanic.**, **GRAPH.**, **Petr.**

CRACKS, fissures

- Painful; feet (3): aq-skook., carc., dys-co.
- Head (4): *aq-carl.*, cupr-ar., **Petr.**, **Ruta.**
- Burning, hands (4): aq-sanic., **Petr.**, sars., zinc.
- Deep; bleeding, hands (9): aq-sanic., alum., graph., *lepro.*, med., **Merc.**, **NIT-AC.**, **PETR.**, **Sars.**
- Hands; winter (13): alum., **Aq-Sanic.**, **CALC.**, calc-s., carbn-s., **Cist.**, **Graph.**, maland., **Merc.**, **PETR.**, **Psor.**, **SEP.**, **SULPH.**

Corns: Aqua Wiesbaden and Aqua Bartfelder

- CORNS; soft (2): aq-wies., **Sil.**
- CORNS; soft; toes, between (2): aq-wies., **Sil.**
- CORNS; stitching, stinging; night (5): aq-bart., ars., nat-m., rhod., **Sulph.**

Heartburn

Remedies: Aqua Destillata, Aqua Carlsbad, Aqua Sanicula, Aqua Gastein.

HEARTBURN

- Chocolate, after (1): aq-des.
- Spices, condiments, piquant, highly seasoned food, after (1): aq-des.
- Drinks; cold, ameliorate (3): aq-carl., arist-cl., mangi.
- Night (13): aq-des., chin., coc-c., con., conch., dysp-n., *eug.*, ferr-p., kali-bi., **Merc.**, posit., ptel., **Rob.**
- Dinner, after (14): acon., aq-carl., calc-p., croto-t., galph., ham., kali-bi., lyc., **Mag-m.**, merc-i-r., *nat-m.*, **Nux-v.**, sol-n., sulph.

- ERUCTATION; smoking; after (6): aq-sanic., bell., **Calc.**, lac-ac., sel., thuj.

- ERUCTATION; milk, of (11): ant-t., aq-sanic., calc., carb-ac., carb-v., cina, lyc., mag-m., merc., sulph., zinc.
- ERUCTATION; waterbrash; pain, with; stomach, in (14): acet-ac., aq-gast., asaf., bism., bism-n., caps., caust., cic., graph., lyc., nux-v., petr., psor., sulph.
- ERUCTATION; waterbrash; salty (15): aq-carl., bry., calc., **Carb-an.**, **Caust.**, euph., lyc., mag-m., merc., **Phos.**, rhus-t., sep., sul-ac., tarax., verb.

Failure to thrive in children

Compare: Aqua Sanicula with Aethusa cynapium and Abrotanum.

A baby/infant with the symptoms below will be failing to thrive – weight not increasing or losing weight. The list of possible causes is very long and many causes can be cured.

The baby needs investigation by a Paediatrician to form a clear diagnosis which prompts treatment – for example, baby/infant may have egg allergy or intolerance, or cow's milk allergy/intolerance, so baby will only get better if the offending food is stopped or replaced: goat's milk or soya formula milk.

Homeopathic treatment is supportive after full investigation and formal diagnosis.

Stomach

- VOMITING; milk; gushing (3): aq-sanic., **Aeth.**, carc.
- VOMITING; milk; after; mother's; nursing, directly after (5): **AETH.**, **Ant-c.**, aq-sanic., ip., **Sil.**
- VOMITING; milk; curdled; lumps, large (5): **Aeth.**, aq-sanic., calc., past., **Valer.**
- VOMITING; sleep; before (8): **Aeth.**, ant-t., aq-sanic., bell., croto-t., **Cupr.**, cycl., **Nat-m.**
- VOMITING; projectile (12): acon., *aeth.*, apom., aq-sanic., **BELL.**, *cupr.*, dys-co., op., phos., thyr., **VERAT.**, verat-v.

> ⚠ Projectile vomiting in a baby requires urgent investigation by admission to hospital – baby may have pyloric stenosis and require surgery.

- APPETITE; wanting; children, babies, in (12): alum., aq-sanic., bar-c., calc., cina, **Gnaph.**, lac-d., lac-h., lyc., nat-p., sac-alb., tub.

Sleep

- FALLING asleep; vomiting, after (6): **Aeth.**, ant-t., aq-sanic., bell., cupr., nat-m.
- SLEEPINESS; vomiting; after (17): **Aeth.**, ant-c., **ANT-T.**, apoc., **Apom.**, **Aq-Sanic.**, ars., *bell.*, chin-ar., cupr., cycl., dig., **IP.**, kali-bi, strep-s., verat., vip.

Abdomen

- ENLARGED; children; emaciation, with (8): **Abrot.**, **Aq-Sanic.**, **Bar-c.**, **CALC.**, hydrang., plb., **Sars.**, **Sil.**

Extremities

- EMACIATION; lower limbs; children, in (3): aq-sanic., **Abrot.**, **Arg-n.**

Neck

- WRINKLED, hanging in folds (5): **Abrot.**, **Aq-Sanic.**, **Iod.**, **Nat-m.**, **Sars.**

Generalities

- WEAKNESS; assimilation, from imperfect (10): alet., alst-c., **Alst-s.**, **Alum.**, **Aq-Sanic.**, **Calc.**, **CALC-P.**, **Nat-m.**, **Sep.**, **Sil.**

Exhaustion – mind – cognitive

Remedies: Aqua Sanicula, Aqua Hochstein, Aqua Carlsbad and Aqua Taosca.

- FORGETFULNESS; details, for (3): aq-sanic., cadm., falco-p.
- FORGETFULNESS; work unfinished, leaves, starts on something else (5): aq-sanic., bac., kali-c., kali-p., *med.*
- FINISH a task, does not, starts another (6): aq-sanic., bac., kali-c., kali-p., lach., med.
- FINANCE; inaptitude for (6): aq-hoch., ars., cypra-e., lyc., puls., **SIL.**
- CONFUSION of mind; motion; ameliorates (5): **Ant-t.**, *aq-carl.*, arg-n., ferr., ferr-p.
- NEGLECTS; everything (6): am-c., *aq-hoch.*, bar-c., caust., tell., ytte.
- BUSINESS; neglects his (9): *aq-hoch.*, *cassi-s.*, lac-lup., lim-b-c., opun-v., ptel., salx-f., **Sulph.**, ytte.
- FORGETFULNESS; Time, for (9): *acon.*, aq-taosc., bamb-a., cath-a., falco-p., **LACH.**, mand., merc., tax.

Exhaustion – body

Remedies: Aqua Wildbad, Aqua Marina, Aqua Hochstein, Aqua Carlsbad, Aqua Franzensbad, Aqua Hall, Aqua Taosca.

Generalities

- LIE down; inclination to; back, on (3): aq-wild., **Phos.**, plut-n.
- WEAKNESS; sudden, paroxysmal; walking, from (4): aq-wild., carb-v., con., sabad.
- WEAKNESS; Rest; ameliorates (12): achy., aq-wild., aran., atista, **BRY.**, gink., hydrog., mag-c., nat-m., nat-n., stann., uran-n.
- MONONUCLEOSIS, after effects of (11): ail., aq-mar., aq-hoch., bar-c., bar-m., calen., carc., crot-c., foll., gali., *thuj.*

Eyes

- WEAKNESS; writing, while (4): aq-carl., bell., **NAT-M.**, **Sep.**

Extremities

- HEAVINESS, weariness: knees; walking; after (5): aq-wild., berb., calc-s., ignis, ruta.

Exhaustion – mind – emotional – overwhelm

Remedy: Aqua Sanicula.

- SADNESS; Fear, with; evil, of impending (5): aq-sanic., **Aur.**, calc., **Caust.**, **KALI-I.**
- SADNESS; menses; ameliorates (8): aq-sanic., arist-cl., **CYCL.**, **Lach.**, macrin., nat-m., **Stann.**, **Zinc.**
- WEEPING, tearful mood; pregnancy, in (9): apis, aq-sanic., ign., lach., **Mag-c.**, nat-m., puls., sep., stann.
- WEEPING, tearful mood; children, in; waking (9): acon., aq-sanic., bell., **Ign.**, lyss., **Med.**, merc., nux-v., sulph.

Remedy: Aqua Hochstein.

- GRIEF; financial loss, from (8): *aq-hoch.*, **Arn.**, ars., **Aur.**, mangi., **Mez.**, pras-o., **Psor.**
- SUICIDAL disposition; love disappointment, from (8): ant-c., aq-hoch., **Aur.**, **Bell.**, **Caust.**, **Hyos.**, plut-n., **Staph.**
- SADNESS; weather; cloudy, in (18): aloe, alum-s., **Am-c.**, aq-hoch., bac., calc-i., *calc-m.*, euro-p., gado-n., germ., harp., lap-c-b., lyc., pall., phos., plat., salx-f., sep.

Chloasma Gravidarum and Aqua Sanicula

Share and Compare: Aqua Sanicula with Sepia and Carbo animalis.

In the old homeopathy books there is a section "Compare" with other remedies – it is the level of share rubrics and compare remedies = Share and Compare in this book. Most readers will know Sepia as having Chloasma

Gravidarum as a symptom in pregnancy, some will know Carbo animalis also has this and I wish all readers to know that Aqua Sanicula has this symptom also. We all look at rubrics and our eyes see the whole rubric but our mind edits out what we do not know – it's called the availability bias.

Face

- YELLOW; saddle across; cheeks (4): aq-sanic., **Carb-an.**, ictod., **SEP.**
- YELLOW; saddle across; nose (8): aq-sanic., carb-an., chel., lyc., op., **SEP.**, sulph., tril.
- SADDLE across nose (10): aq-sanic., **Carb-an.**, chel., ictod., lyc., op., **SEP.**, sulph., syph., tril.
- BROWN; nose (8): aq-sanic., **Aur.**, **Carb-an.**, **Lyc.**, **Op.**, **SEP.**, **Sulph.**, **Syph.**

Breast Sensitivity, Pain and Tumours

Remedies: Aqua Hall, Aqua Teplitz, Aqua Skookum Chuck.

Compare with: Phytolacca decandra, Conium maculatum and Asterias rubens.

Most readers will know Phytolacca decandra, Conium maculatum and Asterias rubens as 3 remedies good for breast symptoms or pathology, some will know Phytolacca as good for breast feeding problems like abscess or mastitis, some will know Conium maculatum and Asterias rubens for cancer breast, and I wish all readers to know that these 3 Aqua have lots of breast symptoms too.

Chest

- SENSITIVE; mammae; nipples; touch of clothing aggravates (3): aq-hall, cast-eq., **Helon.**
- PAIN; stitching; needles, as from; mammae; right (2): adam., aq-tep.
- PAIN; stitching; needles, as from; mammae (9): adam., aq-tep., carb-an., con., grat., iod., kali-bi., ol-an., plb.
- PAIN; burning, smarting; mammae; nipples; left (6): aq-hall, sac-l., **Senec.**, **SIL.**, spira., zinc.

- TUMOURS; painful, mammae (9): aq-tep., berb-a., **Brom.**, calc-i., **Chim.**, **Con.**, phase., **Phyt.**, **Sil.**
- TUMOURS; mammae; right (9): aq-tep., aster., bell., carc., con., lap-be-e., phel., *phyt.*, psor.
- TUMOURS; mammae; left (11): aq-skook., aster., brom., calc-f., calc-p., chim., con., iod., lach., phyt., psor.

Unresolved Grief

Remedies: Aqua Marina, Aqua Hochstein, Aqua Carlsbad and Aqua Taosca can be considered for unresolved grief in the same way that you may consider Ignatia amara, Natrum muriaticum and Phosphoric acidum.

- GRIEF; resigned (4): aq-mar., clem., erb., erb-o.
- GRIEF; prolonged (11): aq-mar., carc., **Caust.**, **Gels.**, **IGN.**, **Kali-br.**, **Lach.**, **Nat-m.**, **Ph-ac.**, phos., thul-m.
- SLEEPLESSNESS; grief, after (14): *aq-hoch.*, aur., carc., **COLOC.**, **Gels.**, graph., **Ign.**, **Kali-br.**, lach., **NAT-M.**, op., **Sulph.**, uran., zinc-val.
- DREAMS; grief (10): all-c., alum., *amet.*, aq-carl., arist-cl., *ars.*, caust., *cyg-c.*, ros-g., stront-c.

Head

- PAIN, headache; grief, after (14): *aq-hoch.*, **Aur.**, **Calc.**, epip., **IGN.**, lact., **Nat-m.**, op., par., **PH-AC.**, **Phos.**, pic-ac., **Puls.**, **STAPH**.

Heart and circulation

- PAIN; heart region; grief, after (17): aq-taosc., bani-c., **Cact.**, camph., choc., dig., **Gels.**, **Ign.**, lach., lap-be-e., lil-t., nat-m., ol-an., puls., pyrus, sac-l., seq-s.

Rectum

- DIARRHOEA; grief, after (11): *aq-hoch.*, calc-p., **Coloc.**, **Gels.**, **Ign.**, **Kali-br.**, merc., op., **Ph-ac.**, *staph.*, sulph.

Sleep Disruption

Remedies: Aqua Kissingen, Aqua Hochstein, Aqua Wiesbaden, Aqua Gastein, Aqua Sanicula, Aqua Lippspringe and Aqua Hall.

- ANGUISH; night; waking, on (4): aq-kiss., kali-br., **Nat-s.**, **Nux-v.**

Sleep

- RISE; must; sleeplessness, from (5): aq-hoch., con., **Nux-v.**, phos., **Rhus-t.**
- WAKING; frequent; restlessness, with (8): aq-kiss., aran., haliae-lc., **Lach.**, latex, m-aust., nicc., **Puls**.
- SLEEPLESSNESS; wide awake (10): aq-hoch., aur., calc., cham., chin., coff., gels., kali-i., sulph., valer.
- SLEEPLESSNESS; pain, with; throat, in (5): *aq-hoch.*, atra-r., kalm., merc-pr-r., methylp-h.
- SLEEPLESSNESS; heat; during; dry (7): aq-wies., **Caust.**, chin-s., clem., **Graph.**, nit-ac., **Thuj.**

- SLEEPLESSNESS; diarrhoea, in (11): aq-gast., bor., **BUFO, Coloc.**, cuph., **Dulc.**, kali-n., merc., **Merc-c., Nat-s., PHOS.**
- SLEEPLESSNESS; hunger, fasting, from (11): abies-n., ap-g., **Aq-Sanic., Chin., Cina, IGN., Lyc., Phos.**, psor., sulph., **Teucr.**
- WAKING; tickling in larynx, from (2): aq-lipp., **COC-C.**
- WAKING; pain, from; chest, in (11): aq-hall, **Bor.**, both-a., chin-s., cit-l., merc-i-r., **Phos.**, rhus-v., sabad., soph-m., **Squil.**
- WAKING; pain, from; back, in (12): ang., aq-lipp., **Bry.**, carc., chion., cinis-p., helo., holm., hom., hydr., plut-n., sel.

Stomach

- APPETITE; ravenous, canine, excessive; sleep, prevents (10): abies-n., aq-sanic., **Chin., Ign., Lyc.**, nat-c., **Phos.**, psor., **Sil., Teucr.**

Earwax

Remedy: Aqua Wiesbaden.

Petroleum is a commonly indicated remedy for earwax problems. When you consider Petroleum, also consider Aqua Wiesbaden.

Ears

- WAX altered; soft (5): aq-wies., *kali-c.*, **Petr.**, sel., sil.
- WAX altered: brown (6): aq-wies., calc-s., con., *irid.*, **Mur-ac., Petr.**
- WAX altered; hardened (11): **ALL-S.**, aq-wies., con., elaps, lach., **Mur-ac., Petr., PULS.**, sel., *semp., verb.*
- WAX altered; thin (20) : act-sp., *am-m.*, aq-wies., cadm., **Con.**, crot-h., flag-l., **Hep.**, iod., **Kali-c.**, lach., **Merc.**, mosch., **Petr.**, sel., **Sil.**, sulph., **Tell.**, tung., *zinc-o.*

Viral Respiratory Tract Infections

Remedies: Aqua Marina, Aqua Franzesbad, Aqua Vichy Grande Grille, Aqua Sanicula and Aqua Hall.

Coryza

Nose

- CORYZA; sleep; ameliorates (2): aq-mar., thea.
- CORYZA; eating; ameliorates after (3): aq-mar., chir-f., oci-s.
- CORYZA; perspiration; aggravates (2): aq-mar., **Nat-c.**
- CORYZA; motion; aggravates (5): aq-franz., galph., naja-m., nat-m., **Nux-v.**
- CORYZA; cough; after (5): aq-vichy-g., bad., **Bell., Hep.**, *kali-n.*

- CORYZA; eating; while (11): aq-sanic., arge-p., **Carb-an.**, clem., hydrog., mangi., nux-v., plb., **Sep.**, sulph., **TROM.**
- INFLAMMATION; catarrhal; evening (7): adam., ant-t., aq-hall, **Carb-an.**, hydrog., mang., **Puls.**

Eyes

- LACHRYMATION; left; coryza, during (3): **All-c.**, aq-franz., napht.

Tonsils

Remedy: Aqua Marina.

Throat

- PAIN; tonsils; right; night (1): aq-mar.
- PAIN; tonsils; right; eating, after, aggravates (1): aq-mar.
- PAIN; tonsils; right; pressure aggravates (1): aq-mar.
- PAIN; tonsils; night (4): aq-mar., ham., ust., zinc.
- PAIN; tonsils; eating aggravates (4): aq-mar., calc., myris., trom.
- PAIN; tonsils; pressure; aggravates (1): aq-mar. OR ameliorates (1): aq-mar.

Remedy: Aqua Bondonneau.

Throat

- HEAT; tonsils (2): aq-bond., iris.
- PAIN; lancinating; tonsils (9): **Amyg-am.**, aq-bond., chel., cub., **Hep.**, merc-i-f., ran-s., raph., ust.

Remedy: Aqua Sanicula.

Throat

- ULCERS; yellow, tonsils; base (1): aq-sanic.
- ULCERS; yellow, tonsils (5): aq-sanic., calc., **Ign.**, manc., zinc.

Laryngitis

Remedies: Aqua Lippspringe, Aqua Teplitz and Aqua Carlsbad.

Sleep

- WAKING; tickling in larynx, from (2): aq-lipp., **COC-C.**

Larynx and trachea

- LUMP sensation; larynx; swallowing, on (2): aq-sanic., ust.
- PAIN; larynx; swallowing; ameliorates (3): aq-tep., spig., tarax.
- PAIN; raw; larynx; morning (11): aq-carl., calc., **Carb-an.**, **Caust.**, cob., **Iod.**, **Rhus-t.**, **Sil.**, **Stann.**, SULPH., zinc.

- MUCOUS in air passages; tenacious; trachea (7): aq-lipp., aq-tep., **Bry.**, **Cann-s.**, just., **Nux-v.**, vinc.

Aqua and Cough

Remedies: Aqua Sanicula, Aqua Lippspringe and Rumex crispus.

Cough

- TICKLING; lying down aggravates (8): aq-sanic., con., herin., hyos., lap-c-b., morg-g., myric., rumx.
- TICKLING; from; chest, in; sternum, behind (17) : ang., aq-sanic., caust., con., hydrog., **Iod.**, iris, mang., med., oxyg., **Ph-ac.**, polyg., **RHUS-T.**, **Rumx.**, *sep.*, **Verat.**, *zinc.*
- DRY; talking aggravates (18): aq-lipp., atro., bell., **Cimic.**, crot-h., dig., **Hep.**, hist., **Hyos.**, lach., **Mang.**, mang-acet., merc., pitu-a., **Puls.**, **Rumx.**, stann., ther.

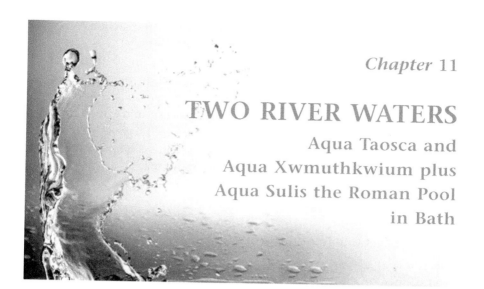

Chapter 11

TWO RIVER WATERS
Aqua Taosca and
Aqua Xwmuthkwium plus
Aqua Sulis the Roman Pool
in Bath

AQUA TAOSCA

Source

The water of the Seven Streams of the Overflowing – in the Burren National Park, Ireland., where there is archaeological evidence of people living since 4,200 B.C.

Content

The Burren is 15 square kilometres of limestone rock formations with hardy wild plants and lichens and some areas of trees. Numerous little crevices within the limestone give sufficient shelter for a variety of alpine plants. The resident fish are eels and 3 spine sticklebacks.[1] No impact from intensive farming or farming chemicals.

The major mineral salts in limestone[2] are: calcium carbonate, calcium bicarbonate and magnesium carbonate. Limestone minerals only dissolve very slowly. It rains often and hard and long in the west of Ireland – the Seven Streams rise fast and overflow. The limestone will erode much more than it will dissolve, but the streams will contain a little calcium carbonate and bicarbonate plus magnesium carbonate.

Proving has been beautifully distilled by Alicia Lee[3] in 2010 and further distilled in 2016[4] with Kingdoms and the Sensation method of Rajan Sankaran and the Periodic Table work of Jan Scholten.

What follows was originally inspired by Alicia's mind map and her generous permission to use as much of it as I needed. I have elected instead to centre this Aqua on rubrics from Van Zanvoort's Complete Repertory 2016[5] with a short section from her original mind map.

Rubrics

Desire to Beget Children and Be a Parent

This is one of the central themes of the Aqua – strong in Aqua Taosca and even stronger in Distilled Water, Aqua Destillata – see chapter 9.

- CHILDREN; desires to; have, to beget, to nurture (8): aq-des., aq-taosc., lim-b-c., lsd, nat-m., *onc-t.*, ox-ac., *plac.*
- CHILDLESS, ailments from being (10): aq-des., aq-taosc., aur., lac-h., lim-b-c., lsd, nat-m., *onc-t.*, ox-ac., plac.
- LOVE; children, for (24): acet-ac., aq-carl., aq-taosc., **Ars.**, chlor., excr-can., ferr-i., gins., **Hep.**, joan., kali-bi., kali-m., lac-eq., lim-b-c., niob., onc-t., ox-ac., ph-ac., phos., *plac.*, plat., sep., verbe-o., *xan.*
- SYMPATHETIC, compassionate, too; children, to (28) : acet-ac., aq-carl., aq-taosc., **Ars.**, chlor., excr-can., falco-p., ferr-i., gins., **Hep.**, ilx-p., joan., kali-bi., kali-m., lac-eq., lant-p., lim-b-c., niob., onc-t., ox-ac., ph-ac., phos., plac., plat., posit., sep., verbe-o., *xan.*

Sensitivity and vulnerability: emotional and cognitive – loss of resilience – overwhelm

Sensitive and vulnerable yet functioning well

- DELUSIONS, imaginations; runs; never before, she can run like (2): agar., aq-taosc.
- DELUSIONS, imaginations; world; world, he is moving in a new (7): aq-taosc., borrel., camph., corv-c., lar-ar., lsd, oplo-h.
- SENSUAL; delights in his own body (1): aq-taosc.
- DREAMS; country; beautiful (8): agath-a., aq-taosc., mel-alt., ol-an., passi., rumx., sile-c., xan.

- DELUSIONS, imaginations; absurd, ludicrous; world is (1): aq-taosc.
- DELUSIONS, imaginations; caves, of (1): aq-taosc.

Loss of Resilience

- DREAMS; exasperation (1): aq-taosc.
- DREAMS; fights; police, with (1): aq-taosc.
- DREAMS; cellars, vaults, crypts (6): aq-taosc., bov., caras., ilx-p., musca-d., uv-lux.
- DELUSIONS, imaginations; footsteps, hears (7): aq-taosc., canth., carb-v., crot-c., **Med.**, **Nat-p.**, soph-m.
- DREAMS; arrested, caught, of being; imprisonment (12): *amet.*, aq-taosc., blatta, borrel., bov., caras., cerv., latex, lsd, *plac.*, posit., stoi-k., taosc.

- FANCIES; lascivious; day and night (3): aq-taosc., chin., dig.
- FIRE; thinks and talks of (5): acan-pl., aq-taosc., bacch-a., **Calc.**, gink.
- FEAR; lightning, of (9): aq-taosc., bell., cycl., dig., dpt, lach., phos., phys., sil.
- FORGETFULNESS; time, for (9): *acon.*, aq-taosc., bamb-a., cath-a., falco-p., **LACH.**, mand., merc., tax.
- INDIFFERENCE, apathy; opinion of others, of (9): agath-a., androc., aq-taosc., bufo, falco-p., neod-f., *stoi-k.*, tax., ulm-c.

Overwhelm

- DELUSIONS, imaginations; mother is cold, hard, cruel (1): aq-taosc.
- FAMILY, aversion to; parents; mother (6): alum-s., aq-taosc., niob., **Posit.**, *scorp.*, **Thuj**.
- FAMILY, aversion to; parents (10): alum-s.,aq-taosc., bor., fl-ac., lat-h., niob., posit., scorp., **Thuj.**, uran.

- GENEROUS, too (11): aq-taosc., bos-s., bros-g., cere-b., electr., nat-m., nux-v., op., staph., sulph., thuj.
- SQUANDERS; money (9): aq-taosc., bac., bute-j., cinis-p., clad-r., culx-p., ind., rhodi., verat.

- KILL, desire to; everyone he sees (3): aids, aq-taosc., hyos.
- RAGE, fury; insults, offenses, after (4): aq-taosc., lat-h., sang., stram.
- RAGE, fury; malicious (11): aq-taosc., **Bell.**, cann-s., choc., cocc., cupr., lyc., mosch., neon, petr., sec.

Sensation as if being in an ancient time

- Looking at the world from a place long ago and close to nature.
- There is no fear about being in this ancient time but there is some anxiety about being able to return to ones actual time. Sitting around a fire with other warriors, the smell of wood smoke and cooking was OK, for a while.

Useful or Unusual Rubrics

Generalities

- AIR; open; desires; seashore, at (4): aq-taosc., euro-o., kali-i., *plac.*
- BATHING, washing; aggravates; hair (3): aq-taosc., succ., tarent.
- EXERCISE, exertion; desires; air, in open (7): ana-i., aq-taosc., **Fl-ac.**, kali-i., lsd, orig., teucr.
- FOOD and drinks; potatoes; desires; fried (14): alum., aq-taosc., cob-n., erb., galeoc-c., glyc-g., hib, lampr-s., nat-m., neod-n., pitu-a., querc-r., sac-alb., tax.
- LIGHTNING, ailments from (13): aq-taosc., bell., crot-h., cycl., dig., dpt, falco-p., lach., morph., **Nux-v.**, *phos.*, phys., sil.

Ears

- PAIN; bathing, washing; aggravates; hair (1): aq-taosc.
- PAIN; bathing, washing; aggravates (3): aq-hoch., aq-taosc., cortico.

Nose

- EPISTAXIS, haemorrhage; walking; aggravates; air, in open (4): aq-taosc., lyc., *m-arct.*, nat-c.
- EPISTAXIS, haemorrhage; walking; aggravates (6): aq-taosc., **Elaps**, lyc., *m-arct.*, nat-c., nat-s.

Smell

- BURNING; clothes (1): aq-taosc.
- SMOKE, of; wood (2): anac., aq-taosc.
- HOSPITAL; like a (2): aq-taosc., crot-c.

Face

- HEAT; burning; lips (3): aq-taosc., arn., psor.

Throat

- TICKLING; right (4): aq-taosc., bapt., dios., vib.

Rectum

- INVOLUNTARY stool; night; bed, in (8): **ALOE**, aq-taosc., **BELL.**, carb-ac., **Plb.**, psor., **Sulph.**, zinc.

Heart & Circulation

- PAIN; heart region; grief, after (17): aq-taosc., bani-c., **Cact.**, camph., choc., dig., **Gels.**, **Ign.**, lach., lap-be-e., lil-t., nat-m., ol-an., puls., pyrus, sac-l., seq-s.

Extremities

- PAIN; hands; tendons (7): aq-taosc., **Brucel.**, ferr-i., led., merl., nat-c., spig., taosc.
- PAIN; ankles; extending; tendo achilles, to (1): aq-taosc.

Share and Compare and Related Remedies

Aqua

Desire to beget children & be a parent: Aqua Destillata & Aqua Hochstein & Aqua Carlsbad.
Fear her condition will be observed: Aqua Marina.
Toothache: Aqua Sanicula.

Solanaceae

Hyoscyamus, Stramonium and Belladonna.

- KILL, desire to; everyone he sees (3): aids, aq-taosc., hyos.
- RAGE, fury; insults, offenses, after (4): aq-taosc., lat-h., sang., stram.
- RAGE, fury; malicious (11): aq-taosc., **Bell.**, cann-s., choc., cocc., cupr., lyc., mosch., neon, petr., sec.

Energy remedies

Positronium, Ultraviolet light, Electricitas, Sol, Magnetus polus arcticus and Magnetus artificialis.

- FAMILY, aversion to; parents; mother (6): alum-s., aq-taosc., niob., **Posit.**, *scorp.*, **Thuj.**
- DREAMS; Cellars, vaults, crypts (6): aq-taosc., bov., caras., ilx-p., musca-d., uv-lux.
- GENEROUS, too (11): aq-taosc., bos-s., bros-g., cere-b., electr., nat-m., nux-v., op., staph., sulph., thuj.
- DREAMS; disappointment (16): aq-taosc., c-di-o., **Cann-s.**, culx-p., echi., harp., hema-h., **Ign.**, latex, perla, posit., rumx., sol, tax., tax-br., ust.

Nose

- EPISTAXIS, haemorrhage; walking; aggravates; air, in open (4): aq-taosc., lyc., *m-arct.*, nat-c.

Smell

- SMOKE, of (9): anac., aq-taosc., bar-c., cor-r., m-art., mand., nic-r., **Sulph.**, verat.

Milks

Lac leoninum, Lac lupinum, Lac delphinium, Lac humanum, Lac maternum.

- DREAMS; stealing, theft; he was (17): alum., aq-taosc., lac-leo., lac-lup.
- DELUSIONS, imaginations; Beautiful, wonderful; things look (17): aq-taosc., hydrog., lac-del., neon, *plac.*, posit., succ., **Sulph**.
- MISTAKES, making; space and time, in (24): aq-taosc., **Cann-i.**, falco-p., **Glon.**, hydrog., *lac-h.*, *lac-mat.*, *mobil-ph.*

Birds

Raven, Whooper Swan, Bald Eagle, Golden Vulture and Peregrine Falcon.

- DREAMS; World; he is moving in a new (7): aq-taosc., borrel., camph., corv-c., lar-ar., lsd, oplo-h.
- DREAMS; Peaceful (9): aq-taosc., coriand., *cyg-c.*, haliae-lc., hippo-k., lac-eq., *mand.*, nux-m., spig.
- FORGETFULNESS; time, for (9): *acon.*, aq-taosc., bamb-a., cath-a., falco-p., **LACH.**, mand., merc., tax.

Nosodes

AIDS, DPT Vaccine, Borrelia burgdorferi, Brucella melitensis, Haemophilis Influenza type B.

- KILL, desire to; everyone he sees (3): aids, aq-taosc., hyos.
- FEAR; Lightning, of (9): aq-taosc., bell., cycl., dig., dpt, lach., phos., phys., sil.
- DELUSIONS, imaginations; World; he is moving in a new (7): aq-taosc., borrel., camph., corv-c., lar-ar., lsd, oplo-h.

Extremities

- PAIN; hands; tendons (7): aq-taosc., **Brucel.**, ferr-i., led., merl., nat-c., spig.

Generalities

- FOOD & drinks; potatoes; desires; fried (14): aq-taosc., alum., cob-n., erb., galeoc-c., glyc-g., hib, lampr-s., nat-m., neod-n., pitu-a., querc-r., sac-alb., tax.

There has been a proving of Limestone from the Burren in 1994 by Nuala Eisig.[6]

Aqua and Limestone Burren (lap-c-b)

Rubrics of 30 remedies or less which contain one or more Aqua plus lap-c-b. The 3 rubrics with Aqua Taosca and Limestone Burren are highlighted with **.

- TIME; timelessness (14): aq-mar., ara-m., brachy-s-p., cann-i., clad-r., cyg-c., lac-lox-a., lap-c-b., *lsd*, mobil-ph., neon, onc-t., spect., tax.
- SADNESS; weather; cloudy, in (18): aloe, alum-s., **Am-c.**, aq-hoch., bac., calc-i., *calc-m.*, euro-p., gado-n., germ., harp., lap-c-b., lyc., pall., phos., plat., salx-f., sep.
- THOUGHTS; persistent; frightful (22) : aeth., **Alum.**, androc., aq-kiss., calc., **Caust.**, hydr., hydr-ac., **Iod.**, kali-br., lac-c., lap-c-b., lyss., op., phos., phys., **Plat.**, **Psor.**, **Rhus-t.**, stram., thea., **Visc.**
- ** FEAR; observed, of her condition being (30): aq-mar., aq-taosc., atro., bamb-a., bar-s., beryl., **CALC.**, cer., cer-c., chel., choc., **Cimic.**, *eryth.*, excr-can., falco-p., galeoc-c., germ., heli., hell., lach., lap-c-b., lsd, lyc., marm-a., neod-s., salv., salx-f., telo-s., terb., terb-o.

Ears

- ** BATHING, washing aggravates (9): *aq-hoch.*, aq-taosc., bor., bufo, cortico., erig., lap-c-b., **Mag-p.**, zinc.

Cough

- TICKLING; lying down aggravates (8): aq-sanic., con., herin., hyos., lap-c-b., morg-g., myric., rumx.
- TICKLING; waking, on (8): alet., aq-sanic., carb-v., ham., her-s., lap-c-b., morg-g., thuj.

Extremities

- ** HEAVINESS, weariness; upper limbs; raising arm aggravates (11): aq-taosc., **Cic.**, *cocc.*, lap-c-b., mag-c., *merc.*, mur-ac., nat-c., paraf., phos., puls.
- PAIN; upper limbs; right; motion aggravates (20): **ACT-SP.**, adam., aego-p., aq-sanic., carc., cassi-f., ferr-p., haliae-lc., hydr-ac., hydrc., **Iris**, lap-c-b., neon, ozone, phos., sang., tarent-c., thymu., ust., verb.

AQUA XWMUTHKWIUM (pronounced 'musqueam').
Also known as Aq-xwm.

Source

Musqueam Creek Water, Musqueam Park, Vancouver, Canada – sacred medicinal water of the native People of the River Grass.

Proving

The proving of the evaporated water by trituration to C7 was carried out by the Coast Salish Trituration. The provers were led by Sandra McLeod[7] – remedy C7/40C.[8]

Rubrics

Sensitivity and vulnerability: emotional and cognitive – loss of resilience – overwhelm

Overactive nervous system.

- Restlessness – desire activity – flitting from place to place – hands restless with a circling motion.
- Sensation as if of great inner energy – not wanting to stay doing any one thing – sensation as if inner jitteriness & as if scattered.
- Sensation as if a cool breeze flowing over body.
- Sensuality – love touch & textures.
- Neuralgic pains moving quickly from place to place – head, abdomen, spine & extremities – alternating with numbness.
- Itching: moves around from place to place – intense continuous itching as if the skin will slough off – feels he might die from the itching – like a horror movie – as if he's covered by spiders & will claw himself to death.

Suppression of emotions and memories – sublimation of libido

- Secrets – the deeper you go the darker it gets.
- Sensation of guilt – as if she has sinned – desire to wash away her sins & become clean again.
- Sensation of shame – desire to forget & deny the past – self medicate with alcohol or recreational or prescribed drugs – hide behind positive new age affirmations.

- Agitation – sensation of frazzled nerves.
- Breasts very sensitive to touch & rubbing.
- Irritability & Anger – comes & goes very quickly – amelioration by inter-ruption – an unforgiving anger.
- Abdominal pain – right lower – causes her to bend over double in agony.
- Bladder: frequent urging to pass urine – painful urination – cystitis.

Grief

- Sorrow – a deep heartache – unforgiving.
- Grief – hidden behind a dam.
- Death – preoccupation with death – thoughts of suicide.
- Angels – ghosts.
- Sour metallic taste in mouth.

Exhaustion – mind & body

- Sensation as if stagnant.
- Sensation as if anaesthetized.
- Sensation as if numbness.

Clinical – Neurological disorders and Skin Eruptions

Vertigo and Neuralgia.

- Vertigo – sensation as if on a small boat rocking on the sea – seasickness – unbalanced – light headed– slipping – clumsy – uncoordinated.
- Neuralgic pains – short, sharp, stabbing in: ovaries, spine, extremities, head, abdomen – in abdomen causing her to bend double – right sciatica – with itchy spine.

Skin

- Sensation as if skin will slough off.
- Eruptions with intense itching & formication – as if covered in spiders & will claw himself to death.
- Slow healing of cuts & wounds.

References

1 Burren National Park website. *Some of the known fish species that inhabit the water systems in the Burren National Park.* National Parks of Ireland. Available online at: https://www.burrennationalpark.ie/gallery-wildlife/fish (Accessed 6th July 2021.)
2 Anon. *Limestone.* Wikipedia, Wikipedia Foundation, 2021. Available online at: https://en.wikipedia.org/wiki/Limestone (Accessed 8th July 2021.)
3 Lee A, *Homeopathic Mind Maps Remedies Animal Kingdom.* Auckland: Moozoonsii Publishing, 2010. pp 87–1119.

4 Lee, A. *Homeopathic Mind Maps. Vol 2. Mineral Kingdom*, 2016 (8th edn), Kandern D: Narayana Verlag, 2016.

5 Van Zandvoot, R. *Complete Repertory*. Leidschendam NL: Institute for Research in Homeopathic Information and Symptomatology, 1994, & *The Netherlands Repertory* 2016. (Accessed via MacRepertory version 8.0.)

6 Eising, N. Limestone Burren. *Provings* (Vol 2). Haarlem: Emryss, 1994. pp 175–223.

7 McLeod S. *The Homeopathic Trituration Proving of Musqueam Creek Water (Aqua XwMuthkwium) Neurological Transformation: Cleansing the Brain of Emotional & Physical Trauma*, 2011. Available online at: https://tinyurl.com/3c8w95rd (Accessed 20th September 2021.)

8 Anon. The Homeopathic Trituration Proving of Musqueam Creek Water (Aqua XwMuthkwium). Neurological Transformation: Cleansing the Brain of Emotional & Physical Trauma. Little Mountain Homeopathy website. Available online at: https://tinyurl.com/3c8w95rd (Accessed 20th September 2021.)

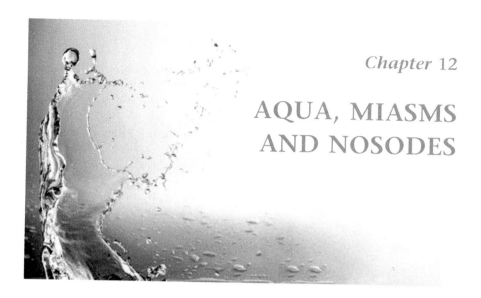

Chapter 12

AQUA, MIASMS AND NOSODES

All of us practising homeopathy appear to be stuck using the word "miasm". What we now mean by miasm no longer bears any resemblance to the dictionary definition. I call on the great ones of homeopathy who write books and teach all over the world and the education committees of ECH and LMHI to work together to give us a short set of sentences and perhaps an acronym to replace it.

I offer a beginning:

- The Vital Force initiates and maintains symptoms for good purpose.
- Some symptoms can be arranged into clusters/groups/sets.
- Some of these symptom sets are required for diagnosis – common, pathological symptoms.
- Some have modalities and sensations and are required to find the most similar remedy.
- Some resemble symptoms of a nosode, for example: aggravation of symptoms from sunset to sunrise.

The Aqua with the widest miasmatic spread of symptoms and related remedies are Aqua Sanicula, Aqua Marina and Aqua Skookum Chuck. Many Aqua remedies have Clinical Rubric Clusters in more than one miasm.

Aqua Sanicula and the 5 major miasmatic nosodes

Generalities

- FOOD and drinks; ham; desires; fat (6): **Aq-Sanic.**, calc-p., **Carc.**, **Card-b.**, **Mez.**, **Tub.**

Stool

- WASH off, odour difficult to (5): aq-carl., **Aq-Sanic.**, **Psor.**, rheum, **Sul-ac.**, **SULPH.**

Rectum

- MOISTURE; fish brine smell (5): aq-sanic., **Calc.**, hydrog., **Med.**, thuj.

Face

- BROWN; nose (8): aq-sanic., **Aur.**, **Carb-an.**, **Lyc.**, **Op.**, **SEP.**, **Sulph.**, **Syph.**

Extremities

- CRACKS, fissures; deep; bleeding, hands (9): alum., aq-sanic., graph., *lepro.*, med., **Merc.**, **NIT-AC.**, **PETR.**, **Sars.**

Other Aqua and the Psoric Miasm

Psora Keywords

- Struggle and effort, lifelong, discomfort, hope, stuck.

Aqua words Psora

- Freezing, melting, snowing, drizzle, shower, rain, trickle, paddling, swimming.

Aqua Rubrics Psora

- GRIEF; financial loss, from (8): *aq-hoch.*, **Arn.**, ars., **Aur.**, mangi., **Mez.**, pras-o., **Psor.**

Ears

- ERUPTIONS; moist; sticky, behind (5): *aq-sanic.*, **Caust.**, dys-co., **GRAPH.** *Psor.*

Nose

- COLD easily, takes (10): apoc., aq-gast., gua., kali-c., lem-m., merc., **Psor.**, silphu., *teucr.*, *tub.*

Perspiration

- PARTS; touching (5): aq-sanic., lach., merc-s., nicc-s., **Psor.**

Vertigo

- DEBAUCHERY, after (4): aq-gast., **Carb-v.**, coriand., nux-v.

Aqua and the Sycotic Miasm. All Aqua remedies? YES

Sycosis Keywords

- Fixed, avoid, hidden, accept.

Aqua words Sycosis

- Glacier, iceberg, aquifer, puddle, fog, mist, moat.

Aqua Rubrics Sycosis

- WEEPING, tearful mood; children, in; waking (9): acon., aq-sanic., bell., **Ign.**, lyss., **Med.**, merc., nux-v., sulph.
- DELUSIONS, imaginations; Footsteps, hears (7): aq-taosc., canth., carb-v., crot-c., **Med.**, **Nat-p.**, soph-m.

Rectum

- MOISTURE; fish brine smell (5): aq-sanic., **Calc.**, hydrog., **Med.**, thuj.

Generalities

- BATHING, washing; ameliorates; sea, in (5): aq-mar., chir-f., hema-h., kali-i., **Med.**

Aqua and the Cancer Miasm

Cancer Miasm Keywords

- Control, perfection, compassion, lifelong effort beyond endurance.

Aqua words Cancer Miasm

- Clear, clarity, crystal, pure, spring, sparkling, pellucid, rainbow, snowflake.
- Current, reflection, still, calm, neutral, buoyant.
- Reverence, repentance, absolution.

Aqua Rubrics Cancer Miasm

- ANXIETY; house or room; aggravates; closed (5): aq-carl., carc., elaps, hist., sulph.
- MISFORTUNE; others, of, aggravates (7): aq-carl., carc., caust., **Coloc.**, corv-c., enal-c., **Tarent.**

Mouth

- PAIN; palate; drinks; hot aggravate (3): aq-sanic., carc., chim.

Stomach

- VOMITING; milk; gushing (3): aq-sanic., **Aeth.**, carc.

Back

- GOOSE flesh (6): aq-sanic., calc-ar., carc., electr., plut-n., **Sarr.**

Aqua and the Tubercular Miasm

Tubercular Miasm Keywords

- Oppression, suffocation, hectic activity to break free, burn-out, bleeding.

Aqua words Tubercular Miasm

- Simmer, boil, pressure, gushing, geyser.

Aqua Rubrics Tubercular

Generalities

- WIND; desire to be in (7): androc., aq-mar., caul., herin., hydrog., *irid.*, **Tub.**
- WEATHER; windy, stormy; ameliorates; cold (5): aq-sanic., **Arg-n.**, lat-h., mur-ac., **Tub.**

FOOD and drinks

- Milk desires; cold; icy (4): **Aq-Sanic., Phos., Rhus-t., Tub.**
- Ham; desires; fat (6): **Aq-Sanic.**, calc-p., **Carc., Card-b., Mez., Tub.**

Aqua and the Syphilitic Miasm

Syphilis Miasm Keywords

- Hopeless despair, degeneration, destruction.

Aqua words Syphilis Miasm

- Erosion, corrosion, dissolved, evaporated.

Aqua Rubrics Syphilitic Miasm

Eyes

- INFLAMMATION; cornea, keratitis; bath, cold, ameliorates (2): aq-mar., **Syph.**

Face

- DISTORTION; one-sided (6): aq-tep., *hyos., merc., nux-v.*, **Syph.**, tell.
- BROWN; nose (8): aq-sanic., **Aur.**, **Carb-an.**, Lyc., **Op.**, **SEP.**, **Sulph.**, **Syph.**

Rectum

- DIARRHOEA; seashore, at (6): aq-mar., **Ars.**, bry., corv-c., **Syph.**, vip.

Aqua and the Leprosy Miasm

Leprosy Miasm Keywords

- Despised, cast out, unclean.

Aqua words Leprosy Miasm

- Stale, stagnant, bog, effluent, sewage.

Aqua Rubrics Leprosy Miasm

Extremities

- CRACKS, fissures; deep; bleeding, hands (9): alum., aq-sanic., graph., *lepro.*, med., **Merc.**, **NIT-AC.**, **PETR.**, **Sars**.
- CRACKS, fissures: feet; soles (9): acan-pl., anac-oc., **Aq-Skook.**, arist-cl., ars., bac., *lepro.*, maland., merc-c.

Clinical

- SARCOIDOSIS (19): aq-mar., aran-ix., asar., beryl., hip-ac., hist., kres., *lepro.*, lyc., mand., nat-ar., parat., parathyr., pin-s., puls., thiop., tub., tub-m., v-a-b.

Aqua and A.I.D.S. Miasm

A.I.D.S. Miasm Keywords

- Contamination through barriers.

Aqua words AIDS miasm

- Seep, permeate, contaminate.

Aqua Rubrics AIDS miasm

- DREAMS; hopeless (4): acan-pl., aids, aq-mar., lac-lox-a.
- KILL, desire to; everyone he sees (3): aids, aq-taosc., hyos.
- ESTRANGED; husband, from her (5): aids, aq-hoch., culx-p., hydr-ac., *thuj.*

- HURRY, haste; time to arrive, for the appointed (10): aids, alum-s., aq-mar., **ARG-N.**, arist-cl., carc., culx-p., cupr., onc-t., ulm-c.

Face

- ERUPTIONS; rash; chin (8): aids, am-c., aq-mar., aq-tep., coriand., **Dulc.**, nic-r., syph.

Mouth

- PAIN; palate; left (3): aids, allox., aq-mar.

Teeth

- PAIN, toothache; extending; nose, to (10): aids, aq-sanic., bar-c., *calc.*, **CAUST.**, cham., eupi., hyos., ip., rhus-t.

Kidneys

- PAIN; extending; back, to (9): aids, aq-hoch., **BERB.**, chol., equis., graph., lac-d., **Solid.**, thymol.
- PAIN; cutting; region of (15): aids, aq-bond., chel., coc-c., germ., **Ipom.**, menth-pu., myric., plb., sapin., scut., solid., **Staph.**, tarent-c., zinc.

Extremities

- CRAMPS; toes; left (5): aids, aq-kiss., brass., lach., v-a-b.
- STIFFNESS; shoulders; left (7): aids, aq-tep., bamb-a., guai., pull-g., salx-f., sep.

Aqua and the Acute Miasm

Acute Miasm Keywords

- Extreme, panic, now or never, life or death.

Aqua words Acute Miasm

- Flooding, drowning, tsunami.

Aqua Rubrics Acute Miasm

- FRIGHT, fear aggravates, ailments from; accident, from sight of an (5): **ACON.**, *aq-hoch.*, **Calc.**, carb-v., **OP.**
- ANXIETY; orgasm of blood, with (12): **Acon.**, aloe, **Am-m.**, aq-gast., **Bar-c.**, carb-an., chel., merl., nit-ac., plb., **Puls.**, **Sep.**

Perspiration

- PARTS; not lain on (7): **Acon.**, **Aq-Sanic.**, **Benz.**, calc., **Nux-v.**, **Sil.**, **Thuj.**

Face

- HEAT; rage, in maniacal (10): **Acon.**, aq-carl., **BELL.**, kali-c., lach., lyc., merc., op., puls., **Verat.**

Aqua and the Malaria Miasm

Malaria Miasm Keywords

- Stuck and harassed.

Aqua words Malaria

- Turbulent, torrent, sinking.

Aqua Rubrics and the Malaria Miasm

Extremities

- PAIN; rheumatic; lower limbs; motion aggravates (6): aq-wies., daph., kali-m., malar., squil., vario.

INDEX